MENTORING AND PRECEPTORSHIP

Other books of interest

REFLECTIVE PRACTICE IN NURSING
The Growth of the Professional Practitioner
Edited by A.M. Palmer, S. Burns and C. Bulman
0–632–03597–8

EXPANDING THE ROLE OF THE NURSE
The Scope of Professional Practice
P. Wainwright and G. Hunt
0–632–03604–4

MENTORING AND PRECEPTORSHIP

A Guide to Support Roles in Clinical Practice

ALISON MORTON-COOPER
MEd, RN

and

ANNE PALMER
BEd (Hons), RN, RM, RNT

OXFORD
BLACKWELL SCIENTIFIC PUBLICATIONS
LONDON EDINBURGH BOSTON
MELBOURNE PARIS BERLIN VIENNA

© 1993 by Alison Morton-Cooper &
Anne Palmer

Blackwell Scientific Publications
Editorial Offices:
Osney Mead, Oxford OX2 0EL
25 John Street, London WC1N 2BL
23 Ainslie Place, Edinburgh EH3 6AJ
238 Main Street, Cambridge,
    Massachusetts, 02142, USA
54 University Street, Carlton,
    Victoria 3053, Australia

Other Editorial Offices:
Librairie Arnette SA
2, rue Casimir-Delavigne
75006 Paris
France

Blackwell Wissenschafts-Verlag GmbH
Düsseldorfer Str. 38
D-10707 Berlin
Germany

Blackwell MZV
Feldgasse 13
A-1238 Wien
Austria

First published 1993

Set by DP Photosetting, Aylesbury, Bucks
Printed and bound in Great Britain by
Hartnolls Ltd, Bodmin, Cornwall

DISTRIBUTORS
Marston Book Services Ltd
PO Box 87
Oxford OX2 0DT
(*Orders*: Tel: 0865 791155
        Fax: 0865 791927
        Telex: 837515)

USA
Blackwell Scientific Publications, Inc.
238 Main Street
Cambridge, MA 02142
(*Orders*: Tel: 800 759-6102
        617 876-7000)

Canada
Times Mirror Professional Publishing,
Ltd
130 Flaska Drive
Markham, Ontario L6G 1B8
(*Orders*: Tel: 800 268-4178
        416 470-6739)

Australia
Blackwell Scientific Publications Pty Ltd
54 University Street,
Carlton, Victoria 3053
(*Orders*: Tel: 03 347-5552)

British Library
Cataloguing in Publication Data

A Catalogue record for this book is
available from the British Library

ISBN 0-632-03596-X

Library of Congress
Cataloging in Publication Data
Morton-Cooper, Alison.
    Mentoring and preceptorship: a guide
to support roles in clinical practice/
Alison Morton-Cooper and Anne Palmer.
        p.   cm.
    Includes bibliographical references
and index.
    ISBN 0-632-03596-X
    1. Mentors in nursing.   2. Nursing—
Study and teaching (Preceptorship)
3. Mentors in nursing—Great Britain.
4. Nursing—Study and teaching
(Preceptorship)—Great Britain.
I. Palmer, Anne.   II. Title.
    [DNLM: 1. Education, Nursing—
methods.   2. Preceptorship.
3. Mentors.   WY 18.5]
RT86.45.M67   1993
610.73'071'55—dc20
DNLM/DLC   93-19829
for Library of Congress   CIP

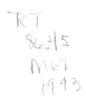

This book is dedicated to
Stan Holder OBE, FRCN
the 'mentor's mentor'
in affectionate recognition of his vision,
support and friendship

Contents

Foreword by Professor Margaret F. Alexander   **xi**

Prcfacc   **xIll**
     Support roles and the new NHS   xiii

Acknowledgements   **xvii**

Glossary of Support Roles   **xix**

1   Creating a Supportive Learning Environment   **1**
     The nature of learning   1
     Context, experience and the learning process   5
     Demands for new learning: the learning agenda   8
     The education of equals   24
     References   25

2   Introduction to Support Roles   **29**
     Why support systems are needed   29
     The changing working culture   29
     The changing UK health service   30
     The case for support systems   33
     Learning support   34
     Emotional support   35
     General support and development framework   36
     Support and development for the student   38
     Peers and peer groups   40
     The roles and responsibilities of academic advisers   41
     Personal tutors   42
     Setting the scene: supervision and facilitation   43
     Nursing – confusion in roles   45
     Coaching in health care   46

The roles and responsibility of the facilitator–coach   47
Assisting with critical reflection   47
Selection criteria for support roles – disabling and enabling 49
    strategies
References   53

3 Mentoring   **56**
What is mentoring?   56
Origins   57
Mentoring terms   57
Influences   58
The *raison d'être* of mentoring   59
Mentoring challenges   60
The classical mentor   61
Character of the relationship   61
Repertoire of helper functions   62
Personal, functional and relational factors   64
Mutual setting of individual purposes and functions   65
Mentor language, functions and organizational culture   65
Organizational applications in business and education   67
Application to health care   68
Choice and mentoring stages   70
Attributes, qualities and abilities of an effective mentor   72
Qualities for attracting a mentor   74
Benefits and limitations of mentoring   75
Strategies for avoiding toxic mentors   76
Constraints to mentoring   76
Formal mentoring: devising a mentor programme   77
Resources and approaches   80
Mentor–mentoree preparation and support   81
The programme   84
Supporting the mentor   86
Evaluation   86
Mentoring case studies   87
The new community midwife   87
Newly qualified and moving on   87
Mature and keen to care   88
The teacher and mentoring comparisons   89
Classical mentoring: positive returns   89
Case studies: the issues   91
References   94
Recommended reading   97

4   Preceptor Support Systems   **99**

What is preceptorship?   99

What makes preceptorship special?   100

Lessons to be learned from the North American literature 102

The attributes of an effective preceptor   109

Expectations of the preceptor relationship   110

UKCC guidance on preceptor support   114

Preceptor selection and preparation   118

Developing a workable curriculum model for practice   123

A suggested curriculum model of preceptorship for
   clinical practice   125

Learning needs, assessment and preceptor preparation   129

Theoretical underpinnings of the curriculum   134

Introducing preceptorship to clinical practice:
   a clinical resource file   137

References   142

5   The Support Agenda: What's in it for the Patient?   **146**

Steps needed to implement a support system   146

Role comparisons   148

A basis for partnership   152

Issues of quality in learning support: an overview of
   ethical concepts   154

What's in it for the patient?   156

References   158

Postscript by Reginald H. Pyne   **161**

Index   **165**

Foreword

Professor Margaret F. Alexander
Head of Department of Health and Nursing Studies
Glasgow Caledonian University

Vision and pragmatism, idealism and stark reality, from fascinating and relevant historical roots to present day flourishing and critical issues – all of these are integral to this book.

It is a most comprehensive and topical map of the terrain of learning in clinical practice. No features of our current health care and nursing landscape are neglected and all of us who are travellers within it are considered. Indeed, it is the first text which I have seen that addresses and proposes solutions to the learning and support needs of staff at all levels of experience, whether their primary responsibilities lie in clinical practice, education, management or research.

The authors' detailed knowledge of their subject and their understanding of the context shine out from every page – a fine blend of the scholarly and the absolutely practical.

This book creates a crisp clarity which illuminates and dispels the cloud of confusion which currently obscures the concept of mentorship and preceptorship. It does this at a time when that state of confusion is potentially at its most damaging; simply because the climate in which health care and nursing are provided is undergoing unprecedented change. Fundamental values about support and enabling others to learn while practising the art and science of nursing, about commitment and caring, too seldom articulated or critically analysed and certainly never realistically costed, are now under the intense, penetrating spotlight of financial scrutiny in the purchaser/provider, market-orientated health care environment. The accompanying outcome measurement orientation challenges nurses – as it does colleague health care professionals – to prepare sound arguments for the establishment of formal supportive frameworks for continuing professional education which not only maximize the individual's potential and motivation to learn from all aspects of nursing practice, but which are manifestly of benefit to patient care.

The authors rise to this challenge. Their proposed framework, which introduces an interesting new and very apposite role of facilitator/coach, elaborates upon four key areas where learning and development needs are particularly important. These bear repetition here and are:

- at entry to the profession, i.e. as a student,
- at entry to professional practice as a newly-registered nurse,
- at transition period of re-entry and/or change of role, and
- at the stage when the experienced nurse moves into a position of influence in the profession as a whole.

Thus, and most importantly, the authors not only make explicit but legitimate the need for all of us, however long or short our experience, at whatever level of seniority or expertize, to have support and to be enabled to continue our learning.

Their exposition of the various support roles they propose are illuminated, in the case of mentorship, by helpful case histories and, in the case of preceptorship, by an outline core curriculum. It is indeed, as the authors state, a 'blueprint for action'.

Although this book is written primarily for nurses, I was pleased to see that the title did not indicate a unidisciplinary focus. It is a rich source of information for everyone involved in nursing, but is equally relevant to all our colleagues in the health care professions. In fact, it has a wider applicability for all for whom learning from experience is important.

So – 'What's in it for the patient?' (See page 146.) Just as the concept of caring is central to nursing, so the concept of caring for colleagues by sharing our knowledge and experience, by enabling and supporting each other in our learning, is crucial to the improvement of the standards of care which we can offer to our patients and/or clients. Learning is a life-long process – a journey of discovery. 'Keep learning how to learn' is a motto, of unknown origin, given to me when I was very young. It is still in my possession today. This book is about learning how to learn from our practice of caring – whether our current involvement is direct or indirect. Use it to the full – it has lots to say to us, both personally and professionally, but above all in relation to the raison d'etre of nursing, the care of our patients.

Preface

Support roles and the new NHS

This book is intended as a blueprint for action in the setting-up of formal support systems for learning in clinical practice.

The need to address the difficulties faced by staff learning in the workplace, and the problems and constraints encountered by those responsible for making wards and units viable for the clinical teaching of students and staff has never been greater.

Policy decisions regarding health service and nurse education reforms, vocational training, staff skill mix, the working hours of junior doctors and the impact of clinical, organizational and learning audit, all carry profound long-term implications for the quality and content of clinical teaching available to health workers in Britain's National Health Service (NHS).

The proposed statutory requirements for registered nurses, midwives and health visitors to update their knowledge and practice, and to provide evidence to support the maintenance and improvement of their competence, has highlighted the urgent need to provide a systematic continuing education strategy which will not only assist the committed employee, but also offer help and support to those who may not have previously enjoyed any formal post-registration learning activity.

This book is aimed at: all nursing staff in practice settings and education; ward and service managers; qualified staff who have responsibility for assisting in the teaching and learning of staff seconded to their wards or units (and particularly those undertaking preparation for teaching and assessing in the workplace); tutors and lecturers in nursing, medicine, and the professional therapies; community nurses, midwives and health visitors; staff counsellors and continuing educators; staff development specialists, and above all, everyone who is expected to or finds themselves acting as a support or role model to staff at work. Managers and trainers in the independent health sector will also find it very helpful and sympathetic to their needs.

Hard and sometimes painful decisions are already having to be made about where employer investment in continuing education can be justified – and often without any detailed appraisal of what constitutes meaningful learning for practitioners being undertaken.

For some, the time-honoured rituals and traditions of becoming an accepted member of the health professions takes precedence over the considered analysis and evaluation of what helps people to practise competently: about how 'expertise' is actually acquired, and about ways in which the patient and client may ultimately benefit from the shared goals and values of staff working in their presumed best interests.

The politics of teaching and learning and the struggle to achieve equity and access to continuing education resources is an underlying theme of this book. It will perhaps challenge widely-held beliefs about the kind of exemplars and support systems we need in order to promote good practice. It will ask you, the reader, to consider your own values and philosophies about what constitutes a good teacher and role model in clinical practice.

The concepts – even the titles – of mentoring and preceptorship have suffered unevenly from misunderstanding and confusion about what each role can realistically achieve. In a desperate bid to implement policy recommendations, colleges and institutions have attempted to grapple with the introduction and maintenance of support systems in different ways. Some have had extremely positive outcomes; other initiatives have ended in disaster.

It is early days in Britain: such concepts need to be carefully analysed, and their uses in other professional fields and countries examined for their relevance to the British health care scene.

Undoubtedly, there are inherent dangers in attempting to apply or transfer concepts interchangeably when the conditions for teaching and learning in one clinical setting are virtually unrecognizable from those in our own institution or specialism.

Rather than imposing new, ill-fitting and superficial support structures on to outdated ones, we must begin to look at the strengths and weaknesses of existing support mechanisms and systems, and think about how we can make them more responsive to perceived learning and support needs.

The need to plan, cost, document and manage the process of providing learning support to staff at periods of transition from one role to another, or one specialism to another, is vital if we are to provide valid evidence and justification for continued access to very limited resources. The sharing and dissemination of our relative successes is also necessary, so that costly mistakes need not be repeated in human as well as economic terms.

The literature would suggest that traditionally we have not been good at supporting our colleagues in times of trouble or uncertainty at work. High wastage rates and rapid turnover of staff demonstrate graphically the need to clarify our expectations of health care work and roles, and to build the networks needed to strengthen and support the workforce through times of challenge and change.

The chapters that follow will ask you to assess the potential for learning support systems in your own field of practice, and will suggest ways in which the richness of practice and the lessons we learn from it can be conveyed in a creative and supportive way, rather than in the clumsy trial-and-error methods we have endured in the past.

We have based the book on the premise that learning itself is a life-long process, and that we all need friends and colleagues to support us in our journeys from 'novice' to 'expert' levels of practice. It recognizes, too, that 'expertise' is a relative term, and that not all of us will want to equate expertness with seniority in the service.

We hope that this book will serve as a valuable guide and beginning resource; that it will help you to raise issues locally, and uncover some of the potential for support and colleagueship across the wide and varied spectrum of health care employment and practice, whatever your background, experience or clinical environment.

Alison Morton-Cooper and Anne Palmer
March, 1993

Acknowledgements

I should like to take this opportunity to thank everyone who has contributed to my own personal support system during the conception, gestation and finally – delivery – of this book.

My colleagues in the nursing support team at Dudley Road Hospital require a special mention, particularly Carol Ward and Maggie Atherton for their inspirational skills of leadership and innovation at times of enormous challenge in our still-reforming health service. Dr Malcolm Tight, my supervisor in the Department of Continuing Education at Warwick University is to be thanked for staying calm and thereby keeping me sane. My husband Barrie and small son, Alastair, have been especially understanding and supportive through low days and holidays.

I should also like to acknowledge the expertise and help given by our editor Lisa Field; the staff of Westwood Library at Warwick; by Barbara Whitehouse, librarian at Arden House Library, and by all my colleagues at work in the NHS, in publishing, and in the ever-growing network of independent continuing education researchers and practitioners helping to move practice and analysis forward.

Anne Palmer, my former tutor and now partner in publication, has been instrumental in making such consultancy credible.

I should like to acknowledge the kind assistance of Reg Pyne, Margaret Wallace and Heather Williams of the UKCC in helping me to stay ahead of the preceptor requirement, and thank the UKCC for permission to reproduce the preceptor requirement in full.

Alison Morton-Cooper

It is an interesting reflection on the nature of our times that the Hillingdon School of Nursing where I did my initial nurse training and St Mary's School of Nursing, Paddington, where I spent my formative teaching years, no longer exist. They have been reorganized and amalgamated as part of the health service changes. They do however live on in my memory, and in my abilities to accept new challenges without fear or trepidation.

I am grateful to the staff, colleagues, students and patients of both these Institutions and the other areas of the National Health Service, for keeping me motivated and learning over the years. I would particularly like to thank the librarians in the local colleges of health who were kind, courteous and always willing to search for information. Special thanks to John Barrington, who is always ready to assist and prepared to share his world of books and to Lisa Field who shared her creativity and experience.

For my parents, and Jude, Maggie and Alan; thank you for your unconditional love and support; with love and thanks to Margaret Alexander, Eric Evans, Winifred Hector, Chris Gill, Stan Holder, Charlotte Kratz, Catherine McCloughlin, Dilly Millward, Andrea Wilson, Edna Quinn and Mary Waltham for sharing the DNA and showing me the way; and of course to Alison who started in my mentor footsteps, but who now leads the way with preceptorship.

I also wish to express my gratitude to my colleagues on the MA course and the lecturers at the Centre for Higher Education Studies, University of London – in particular Ron Barnett, Robin Middlehurst and Susan Weil, who stimulated my thought processes and halted my 'academic drift'.

Anne Palmer

Glossary of Support Roles

This is not intended to be exhaustive or complete. As considerations and the debate about support roles develop and new understandings emerge so will our interpretations of what is available and on offer. Roles that are currently topical include the following (references cited in Chapter 2):

Assessor: A professionally competent practitioner who is prepared in the skills required to assess the performance of another.

Clinical supervisor: A skilled practitioner who observes, assesses, advises and practises with another to enable him/her to attain professional skills. The degree of supervision should reflect the personal development and competence of the less experienced, learning individual. Butterworth (1992) views clinical supervision as 'an exchange between practising professionals to enable the development of professional skills'. (Butterworth, 1992, p. 12).

Facilitator–coach: A skilled practitioner who provides an understanding of the nature of professional practice, through the provision of learning opportunities and supportive intervention. Facilitating–coaching involves constructive monitoring and feedback of performance to aid learning, self-awareness and personal development, allowing the student to practise effectively.

Mentor: Someone who provides an enabling relationship that facilitates another's personal growth and development. The relationship is dynamic, reciprocal and can be emotionally intense. Within such a relationship the mentor assists with career development and guides the mentoree through the organisational, social and political networks.

Peer, peer pals, buddy: Someone considered a colleague of equal status, forming a collaborative relationship that is mutual and non-competitive. A peer group as a collection of peers can provide an informal, supportive network acting as colleagues and friends.

Preceptor: An identified experienced practitioner with responsibilities for a client group who enhances learning by teaching, instructing, supervising and role modelling.

In UK nursing, this role has been modified to mean a qualified and experienced registered nurse, midwife or health visitor who works in partnership with a (newly) registered practitioner colleague in order to assist and support them in the process of learning and adaptation to their new role (Morton-Cooper, 1993).

Role model: This provides demonstrable behaviour that merits imitation, (Bandura, 1962 & 1987). By observation of the chosen role model's behaviour, an image is formed that can be imitated. Such modelling involves the processes of identification, observation, imitation and the comparison of 'visible experts', (Rawlins & Rawlins, 1983). A role model assists learning by example.

Chapter 1
Creating a Supportive Learning Environment

The nature of learning

> 'Wen you're a married man, Samivel, you'll understand a good many things you don't understand now, but vether it's worthwhile goin' through so much to learn so little, as the charity-boy said ven he got to the end of the alphabet, is a matter o' taste!'
>
> Mr Weller, in Charles Dickens' The Pickwick Papers

In Weller's words, is learning worth the pain? The Greek philosopher Aristotle clearly thought so:

> 'To accustom children to the cold from their earliest years is an excellent practice, which greatly conduces to health, and hardens them for military service. Hence many barbarians have a custom of plunging their children at birth into a cold stream; others, like the Celts, clothe them in a light wrapper only. For human nature should be early habituated to endure all which by habit can be made to endure; but the process must be gradual. And children, from their natural warmth, may be easily trained to bear cold. Such care should attend them in the first stage of life...'
>
> (from The Politics of Aristotle, see Jowett, 1899)

Aristotle's influence on Western education and its traditions has been enormous. His thinking was that a primary aim of education should be to produce a virtuous person, and that education should be a function of the State. He felt the tension about the purpose and value of education, and about whether it should be concerned with moral or intellectual virtue (Ozman & Craver, 1990).

The argument about whether formal education in health care should be concentrated on organizational or personal learning needs is relived daily in our hospitals, colleges and communities – particularly when it comes to assessing the cost/benefits of any financial support.

The notion of enduring hardship in order to make learning worthwhile permeates our initial schooling and education, and for some, leaves a feeling that if learning is fun it can't be *real learning*. Real learning requires a serious and arduous attempt to grapple with things which, at best are foreign to us (like maths and languages), and at worst are dictated to us by those who believe they know better than us what it is we *should* learn.

Theories about what constitutes learning and a valid learning environment have evolved over centuries, although the perspectives and involvement of now familiar disciplines such as psychology and sociology have only emerged in this context since the mid-nineteenth century.

It is interesting to see that some of our contemporary models of clinical teaching and learning – such as one-to-one teaching and case-study methods – are still quite faithful to those expounded by the Graeco-Roman physicians, surgeons and 'midwives' of the pre-Christian era (Nutton, 1992).

We tend to talk about education for health care as a very modern phenomenon, and look for innovatory methods of teaching and learning without perhaps looking in detail at some of the rationales behind the methods used by the early practitioners and philosophers of health care.

Some of their thought processes are very revealing. In an essay on the social history of Graeco-Roman medicine one medical teacher describes 'a good midwife' as 'a paragon of virtue, intelligence, energy and patience, to say nothing of her long fingers and soft hands' (Nutton, 1992, p. 54).

This might be considered amusing now, if it weren't for the disturbing legacy it enjoys in current health care practice. Jane Salvage, the popular nurse journalist who now promotes nursing as part of the World Health Organization wrote the following on the public image of nursing in 1986:

> 'The stereotype nurse is likely to work in a hospital ward caring for surgical patients or others with diagnosed diseases from which they will soon recover, but the NHS actually deals with many other problems. Over half its beds are occupied by people with long term problems caused by old age, mental or physical handicap or mental illness. In romantic novels and comedy films, however, doctors cure diseases, nurses clear up the mess and hold the patient's hand, the patient goes home well, and nurse and doctor celebrate by getting married...'

> (Salvage, 1986, p. 25)

As nurses, therefore, we are comfortable with notions of our being intelligent and energetic, but extremely sensitive to any inference of nursing as an overtly feminine 'virtue', largely because of its perceived close relative – the notion of subservience – where nurses and midwives are perceived as doctors' handmaidens, and therefore secondary to the caring process.

It may be partly for this reason that there is no common practice in the UK for medical and nursing students to be formally taught or undertake learning together, although this is becoming more usual in post-graduate education and training in the NHS (Reigelman *et al.*, 1985).

Mutual suspicion about motives for learning can lead to mis-understanding between beginning professionals about *what* we are expected to learn and *why* we are expected to learn it, leading in turn to value judgements about what constitutes proper learning. This seems a shame, particularly when the potential for sharing values and combining learning opportunities seem great (Pietroni, 1991).

For example, how often have we heard the moans about the medical student who knows all about anatomy and physiology and nothing about the emotional problems associated with illness? How many nurses have been criticized for not knowing one vein or artery from another when it comes to helping a junior doctor insert an intravenous catheter? It's possible that a good many opportunities for learning are lost in clinical practice because of the separatist tendency to teach medical and nursing students as if they had no mutual interest in the care being given or techniques being demonstrated.

In a discussion on the preclinical curriculum in medicine Downie and Charlton (1992) say that there are 'three main aspects to a good doctor: knowledge, skills and a certain humane and wise attitude to patients'. They argue that while knowledge is developed through the curriculum and specialized and continuing medical education, skills are developed through clinical practice. Medical knowledge and skills are developed by means of the study and practice of both medical and social sciences. *Attitudes*, however, are left undeveloped and unquestioned.

Bradby's very enlightening study of the ritualized 'status passage into nursing' (Bradby, 1990) also demonstrates the lengths we go to as an occupational and social group of individuals to avoid addressing some of the very emotional and painful aspects of learning and dealing with the internal conflict brought about by working with people at their most vulnerable and dependent.

Bradby describes 'status passage' as 'the process of change from one status to another', as in moving from a student to a practitioner role. In her study, she examined the emotional effects of undertaking certain aspects of patient care, and discussed their implications for clinical learning (Bradby, 1990). She looked at how patient care was managed in those areas which tend to arouse ambivalent feelings in the career, such as caring for the incontinent patient, the very ill, those with altered body image, the mentally confused, and those who have made a suicide attempt.

Her findings highlighted the lack of preparation students were given for managing or 'coping' with such tasks, and the lack of support they received from trained staff. Supervision of the 'essential care' given to patients by students was not always regarded as important by the trained staff, and often the trained staff did not appear to understand the psychosocial problems experienced by patients.

Bradby concluded that despite beginning clinical practice being considered the most exciting part of entry into nursing, is also provoked anxiety: caring for patients, the *raison d'être* given for entering nursing, was fraught with 'feelings of confusion, anxiety and of being overwhelmed.'

Students in the main had to 'chart their own status passage in providing patient care, with the possibility of providing perfunctory and incorrect care'. She surmised that this might in part be due to the 'busyness' of the ward, but also due to the lack of staff available for direct supervision. Some staff did not consider it important, or perhaps they did not know how, to cope with certain situations either, (which wouldn't be surprising, given their *own* status passage into nursing).

Some nurses were able to adapt their responses; others remained defensive. Those with low self-esteem and high anxiety scores were the most vulnerable:

> 'Theoretical input (on such matters) was minimal, and though clinical teachers helped in one hospital, the main support came from other trainees. It is sad to relate that in some areas of nursing work little seems to have changed since the studies which were published at the end of the 1950s. This may be due to the fact that these areas of care are the taken-for- granted world of the nurse and so are not deemed worthy of special study. In reality, of course, they are the very areas which the trainee nurse must successfully bridge in the transition from lay person to nurse. We ignore them at our peril ...'
>
> (Bradby, 1990, p. 1368)

The totality of the clinical learning environment therefore presents itself regardless of whether or not we value some aspects of it more than others; and whether we consider one form of care provision to be more glamorous or important than any other we experience.

Learning situations abound even in the 'taken for granted world' which we inhabit daily, and even though, when we have qualified and succeeded in charting our way somewhat warily into the ranks or echelons of our chosen profession or occupational group, we still have a tendency to replicate our previous learning experiences.

We expect in-comers to 'prove themselves' sailing by the same waters and overcoming the same fears in the same haphazard and unnecessarily painful ways.

Failure to legitimize and to take responsibility for helping others to learn from difficult experiences in a more structured way may be part of what we mean when we lament the lack of necessary support from our colleagues.

Before being able to provide help, however, we need to recognize and articulate the problem. What constitutes a supportive learning environment and what can we do to bring it about?

To begin with, whether we are talking about a classroom or lecture room situation, or a one-to-one teaching session in a patient's home, there is a need to acknowledge the importance and influence of both *context* and *experience*.

Context, experience and the learning process

The idea that learning can transform us as human beings from passive bystanders to pro-active givers is a popular one in contemporary adult education literature. Mezirow (1990), for example, believes that:

> 'To make meaning means to make sense of an experience; we make an interpretation of it. When we subsequently use this interpretation to guide decision/making or action, then making meaning becomes learning.'

> (Mezirow, 1990, p. 1)

He breaks this down further by saying that we learn differently when we are learning to perform than when we are learning to understand what is being communicated to us. Reflection (for example) enables us to correct distortions in our beliefs and our errors in problem-solving.

In his view, learning may be defined as the process of making a new or revised interpretation of the meaning of an experience, which then guides subsequent understanding, appreciation, and ultimately, action:

> 'What we perceive and fail to perceive and what we think and fail to think are powerfully influenced by habits of expectation that con- stitute our frame of reference, that is, a set of assumptions that structure the way we interpret our experiences.'

(Mezirow, 1990, p. 1)

Mezirow believes that it isn't possible to understand the nature of adult learning or education without recognizing the cardinal role played by these habits in 'making meaning'.

Essentially, what he says is that the 'taken for granted' world alluded to earlier is in fact made up of all our perceptions, beliefs and assump- tions of what constitutes our reality, and that we construct or build it for ourselves on the basis of our past and present experience. We contribute to it or take from it according to our own ideas about such things as right and wrong, social justice, and the individual parts we play in acting out the roles society requires of us.

As adults we don't enter a learning situation as an empty jug needing to be 'filled' with learning, (the so-called 'jug and bottle' or 'empty vessel theory'); rather we come to it with all the preconceptions and feelings of someone who has experienced the transition from child to teenager to adult. We have views about things: about what being 'mature' means, about not being 'silly', about being 'responsible' rather than 'irrespon- sible' (Boud, 1981).

We come laden with value judgements about what is useful in life and what is helpful. Sometimes we choose to rely on others whom we con- sider to be 'expert' in a given subject or area, and trust them to reveal to us and teach us about what is important or valuable in this context from their repertoire of knowledge, skills and attitudes. The doctor–patient relationship is a good example of this, as is the situation of a history tutor preparing a pupil for an 'A'-level exam.

Just as we bring our previous experiences to a learning situation, however, so does the context in which learning is to take place reflect previous experiences. Psychologists and educators have made careful study of the social and climatic conditions appropriate for learning (e.g. Gagne, 1975, Rogers, 1980, Knowles, 1980), and of the impact stages of human development have on our 'readiness to learn' (Cross, 1981; Tennant, 1988).

The 'fixed variables' or immutables of the setting in which we learn are much less easy to define, partly because we do in fact take them for granted. It's hard to imagine a school without classrooms for example, or a hospital without beds.

The treatment room of a GP's surgery or the five feet by ten feet cubicle of an acute hospital casualty department are fixed and unchanging environments for care. Our expectations of what goes on in them are likely to be determined by (1) our previous first- and second-hand experiences, imaginings, and any exposure to such things in the newspapers or on television and (2) (as students of health care) by what we have been led to expect by our colleagues, fellow students, senior staff, patients and lecturers.

The context itself brings with it certain associations and assumptions such as gloom, doom or happiness, depending on our views and personalities. The words or concepts of 'funeral parlour' and 'funfair' may be equally nightmarish to some people, while seeming to represent conceptual opposites or contradictions to others.

When we plan a learning experience, then, we need to remember that both context and experience can promote and inhibit learning from the perspective of the individual learner.

Freedom and responsibility

These concepts, too, may appear to contradict one another. The extent to which we are free to learn what we want to is limited by our motivation for learning. If we want to be accepted as part of a certain group, then we anticipate having to learn the rudiments of the skill first, with a view to becoming competent in that skill, and perhaps (with work and determination), becoming experienced or even an 'expert'.

Novice skiers and cyclists begin this way, as do artists, musicians and writers. But is it legitimate for health professionals to view their practice and professional development in this way? Guidance on how competence or 'fitness for purpose' can be defined sometimes reflects our collective assumptions and what we regard as progression towards 'safe practice'.

Our justification for including certain subjects in a curriculum are found in moral arguments about the nature of care we wish to provide, and the boundaries or limitations made on care provision by our emotional as well as financial resources.

Codes of professional conduct and committee-derived 'ethical guidelines' are attempts at defining boundaries and professional 'freedoms' to practise in a way deemed permissible by those vested with the appropriate authority and wisdom.

Much of the impetus for learning and for change and innovation in health care practice in the UK in recent times has come from government reforms in the provision and meting out of health care resources, and from the recommendations of the various statutory bodies, professional and lay organizations which claim to represent the interests of the state, professionals and patients respectively.

Pressure to conform and perform to given standards is a powerful motivator for continuing learning – because in some instances failure to do either could lead us to fail in our jobs, and fail to meet the expectations of our employers, our patients and, of course, our peers. To fail may mean becoming unemployed or unemployable.

Our freedom to learn as health workers, then, is relative to our ability to justify what is appropriate to learning about health care, and about exactly what it is that we want to achieve by learning. This could be described as freedom to learn with responsibility.

Demands for new learning: the learning agenda

There are some four million trained nurses in the world according to the last official count in 1986. About 15% of these are thought to be working in the developing countries, where over two-thirds of the world's population live. Between 80 and 95% of all nurses spend their working lives in hospitals, which means that most are to be found in urban centres rather than in rural communities. In global terms, as much as 90% of available resources goes into providing institutional health care (Seivwright, 1988).

The theoretical demand for continuing nurse education which responds to changing health needs is therefore virtually limitless.

By this calculation the ratio of qualified nurses, midwives and health visitors in Britain to its general population is roughly 1 to every 88 people (or 0.01% of the population), a disproportionately high figure in relation to the rest of the world (with the possible exception of the USA for which no comparable figures are obtainable).

The extent to which nurses in Britain are 'trained' rather than educated has become a major issue recently, although it is one which continues to be debated from a very insular perspective – i.e. from the point of view of nursing in Britain in the foreseeable future, rather than the more global view of the preparation of nursing leaders in the pursuit of 'Health for All', as described by the World Health Organization in 1979 (WHO, 1979). This does seem a shade ironic given that British nurses have in the past claimed to lead the world in terms of nursing innovation (Leddy & Pepper, 1989).

It would seem to make good sense therefore to balance the educational preparation of nurses with the jobs they are aiming to do.

In developing countries – where an estimation of the level of educational attainment of nursing recruits is unpredictable, and where teaching resources are extremely limited – it may be that the notion of 'training' towards some common principles could be considered a legitimate 'learning outcome'.

The learning priorities for these are of necessity defined by the most pressing problems confronting health workers and local and international relief agencies; whether they be a combination of drought, starvation, diarrhoeal, malarial or typhoid infection; the need for immunization and other primary prevention programmes, or the teaching of basic hygiene measures to stave off epidemic recurrences of infections which have become indigenous to that population.

Westernized or 'first world' countries, on the other hand, have very different expectations of the nurse's role. This is reflected in the diverse demands for health care in westernized societies, demands which have a tendency to be those of the most articulate and not necessarily the most needy because of social class divisions and problems of powerlessness in vulnerable communities (e.g. Townsend *et al.*, 1988).

The expectations of health care provision in Britain and the United States are possibly so wide as to defy any kind of rational, widely applicable definition of preparation for practice in nursing.

Nurse educators and policy-makers in the late twentieth century could be said to have an intractable problem: attempting to provide an education which will equip their students with sufficiently transferable basic skills to enable them to practise (as a beginner at least) in any clinical situation.

Because this expectation has now been recognized as unrealistic in Britain, the challenge has been laid at the continuing educator's door. It is therefore the function of continuing education staff to help practitioners make up the perceived shortfall in terms of their knowledge base and clinical expertise, as well as to help them provide written evidence of their achievements in a form acceptable to their employers.

But what of the growth of education for education's sake in recent years? To what extent must nurses concede to the instrumentalist and humanitarian view of nursing as an altruistic utilitarian self-sacrificing activity? And to what extent are nurses in 'first-world' countries to be allowed to join the growing band of adults who pursue learning for love of learning rather than for its perceived attendant skill-giving properties?

Cross (1981) declares that the learning society is growing because it must. She argues that it would be difficult to live in a society which is changing as rapidly as ours without constantly learning new things:

'When life was simpler, one generation could pass along to the next generation what it needed to know to get along in the world; tomorrow was simply a repeat of yesterday. Now, the world changes faster than the generations, and individuals must live in different worlds during their lifetimes . . .'

(Cross, 1981, p. 1)

She quotes Toffler (1970, p. 14) as saying that most people are 'grotesquely unprepared to cope' and that as the pace of change continues 'mass disorientation' in society may be the result.

Looking closely at the history of the industrialised nations Cross describes the trends which have influenced the evolution of adult education practice, beginning with the concept of the linear life plan, i.e. 'a life pattern in which education is for the young, work for the middle aged, and leisure for the elderly' (Cross, 1981, p. 9).

It was thought that the compression of work activities into the middle years may well have brought about the temptation to push young people back to school and older people into ever-earlier retirement – a position identified by Best and Stern (see Cross, 1981, p. 10) and one which accurately reflects the state of unemployment and social life in Britain in the early 1990s.

Best and Stern's solution to this problem came in the form of an alternative to the 'linear life plan' known as the 'cyclic life plan' (Best & Stern, 1976). The basic purpose of this was to redistribute work, education and leisure across a person's life span. By alternating patterns of study, work and leisure, learning became repeated and 'recurrent', and theoretically a part of everyone's life, rather than a one-off occurrence taking place at the statutory or accepted 'school age'.

The notion of 'sabbatical' or educational 'leave' then came into vogue, but as Cross points out, few employers could be persuaded to afford these practices. Instead, Cross suggests another way to break-up the steady diet of education/work/leisure by moving towards what she describes as the 'blended life plan', by which she means that:

'Work, education and leisure are concurrent, rather than alternating, at all points throughout life.'

(Cross, 1981, p. 12)

Allegiance to the idea of in-service education in Britain may therefore be a manifestation of a similar trend to that described above – although its origins here may be traced back to the adult education movements of the nineteenth century in the form of parish education, worker's educational colleges and various university extension initiatives (Curtis & Boultwood, 1964).

Although the cost-effectiveness of combining work and study is often assumed in the literature it is difficult to find concrete and reliable evidence to support some of the claims made for in-service education on the basis of its *educational value, vis-à-vis* the benefits it brings to employing organizations in the form of greater integration and conformity of employees to stipulated employer-defined objectives.

'Training' tends to define tasks primarily in terms of increasing knowledge and skills, thereby focusing attention on that which is more easily 'programmed'; it doesn't readily take into account the role the learner can play in defining, analysing and resolving his or her own dilemmas outside of narrow pre-defined frameworks (Marsick, 1987).

Dearden (1990) says that the point of learning in vocational training is to secure an operative efficiency: the person will be able to operate the word processor, administer the injection or run the shop. The point of learning under the aspect of education, however, is to secure breadth and depth of understanding, a degree of critical reflectiveness and corresponding autonomy of judgement. He argues that the former can work well where training is liberally perceived (for example, he cites teacher training as a liberal interpretation of training), but the 'illiberally conceived' training could be described as *anti-educational*, by promoting habitual acceptance of authority without any reflection or consideration of possible alternatives (Dearden, 1990, p. 93).

The concept of 'education' can also be reviewed as an emancipatory force which will help oppressed individuals to free themselves from the chains which bind them to their oppressors, largely by a process of action based on critical reflection, which in turn allows people to recognize who or what it is that oppresses them in the first place (Freire, 1972; Glen, 1990).

Such a tension between what is useful to the organization providing the learning, and that which is valued by the learners themselves, is one of the most difficult for us to resolve satisfactorily. Attempts to serve the two by combining the rationales of both training and learning needs, and identifying common areas of interest is one possible answer to this problem – but this is to assume that some common ground is likely to exist, a theory which is not necessarily borne out in practice. In order to try and detect where that common ground might be, however, it is helpful to look at what adult educators have said about the processes of adult learning.

One of the most influential adult educators (in nursing terms) has been Malcolm Knowles, advocate of the concept of 'andragogy', or the 'science and art of what makes adults learn' (Knowles, 1984).

Knowles' famous distinction between the traditional teacher-centred approaches of childhood education, known as 'pedagogy', and that which is primarily adult-centred, described as 'andragogy', appears to have galvanized nurse educators in the mid-1980s to new aspirations, when they began to perceive nursing students as adults and individuals, rather than mass intakes of unthinking, uncritical, uninspiring school-leavers.

The time-honoured didactic traditions of earlier nurse teaching no longer pertained to the better-educated, more self-aware entrant to nursing in the 1980s, and so an alternative to existing teaching and learning methods had to be found.

Although the dividing line between childhood and adult education is a difficult one to assess conceptually (see Davenport, 1993), it is becoming more widely recognized that the nurse who is able to initiate and direct his or her learning in order to function in a world of rapid change is more likely to remain competent in the delivery of a humane and effective service than the nurse who has not acquired those skills (Richardson, 1988 cited in Silcock, 1991, p. 27).

The importance of reflectivity in learning

Mezirow (1983) attributes the human tendency to move towards new perspectives to a collective search for solutions to the 'disorienting dilemmas' confronting us, and essentially as a quest to find meaning in life.

Mezirow believes that 'perspective transformation' (i.e. 'the structure of psychocultural assumptions within which new experience is assimilated and transformed by past experience' (1983, p. 125)) fills an important gap in adult learning theory, by acknowledging the central role played by the function of 'critical reflectivity':

> 'Awareness of *why* we attach the meanings we do to reality, especially to our roles and relationships ... may be the most distinguishing characteristic of adult learning'.

> (Mezirow, 1983, p. 128)

He goes on to differentiate between different types of reflectivity:

- Affective reflectivity, which refers to the way we feel about an activity.

- Discriminant reflectivity, where we identify causes for behaviour, and set these in the context of our reality.
- Judgemental reflectivity, which is our awareness of the value judgements which inevitably colour our perceptions, thoughts, actions and habits in a given situation.

As was suggested earlier, Mezirow concludes that helping adults to construe everyday experience in a way that helps them to understand the reasons for their problems, and so to understand further the options remaining open to them, is part of helping adults to take responsibility for their own decision-making, a process which he believes is 'the essence of education' (Mezirow, 1983, p. 134).

Mezirow's thinking, then, leans heavily towards the Freirian emancipatory school of adult education, but he is also cognisant of Knowles' argument, that adults need to be self directed in their learning if they are to benefit from and appreciate any relevance in that learning (Knowles, 1984).

Many other authors have described the concept of reflectivity in relation to adult learning, notably Dewey (1933), Schon (1983), Kolb (1984), Boud *et al.* (1985), Jarvis (1983; 1987) and Burnard (1988). Dewey, for example, identified one solution to doubt, conflict and obscurity in understanding, by re-producing the concept of 'reflective thinking'.

Dewey advocated a number of possible solutions to problems, such as constructing hypotheses about them which could be tested, the use of data collection, and of reasoning and experimentation with problems. As Jarvis (1987) explains, Dewey did not always expect these approaches to run consecutively, but he did think it was possible to detect a problem solving cycle in these processes:

> 'Dewey suggested certain qualities of mind, such as sensitivity, imagination, the ability to analyse and synthesise and the power to reason, that should be among the qualities of an educated person'
>
> (Jarvis, 1987, p. 87)

Cervero (1992) recently pointed out that Dewey was not the first to observe that learning from practice is meaningful: the Scottish philosopher David Hume once remarked on it, and Aristotle before him.

Cervero also offers three propositions as a basis for the improvement of continuing education for the professions, namely, that:

(1) The goal of professional practice is wise action.
(2) Knowledge acquired from practice is necessary to achieve this goal.

(3)   A model of learning from practice should become the centrepiece
      of systems of continuing education for the professions.

                                                      (Cervero, 1992)

He reminds us that professionals' actions are never value-neutral, and as
such they must be judged as wise within their given ethical framework.
In the case of nurses presumably the UKCC's Code of Conduct is the
ethical framework, acting on behalf of the general public.

Cervero describes the process of 'reflection in action' as the core of
professional artistry, and cites Schon's model of reflection as an action
orientated social process which is developmental, and also allows professionals to reason from general rules about 'problematic cases',
thereby moving on to develop and test new forms of understanding and
action in practice.

The proper use of reflectivity in continuing nurse education is a
legitimate concern of those planning provision in the workplace, as it no
doubt is in colleges and higher education establishments.

Providing the opportunities for 'reflection in action' is becoming more
difficult, however, as the perceived imposition of the supernumerary
student in a one-to-one consultation (such as the 'student' out on-call
with the community psychiatric nurse) is becoming more difficult to
justify to patients, particularly in sensitive and intimate situations.

Whilst it may once have been acceptable to have a student 'tag along'
on the basis of 'learning from Nellie', as the apprentice who had to work
while learning a trade, the presence of a stranger who has no observable
contribution to make to the nurse–patient relationship is less easy to
explain.

Once patients become accustomed to regular visits from students or
qualified staff who are non-participant observers, (either in hospital or in
the community) it is possible that they may subconsciously (or con-
sciously) alter their behaviour towards the nurse who has been allocated
to them for care. Anecdotal experience already suggests that patients
may hide their real concerns until such times as they are able to discuss
the matter in confidence with their nurses.

A report from the National Audit Office highlighted problems
expressed by community health managers in finding appropriately
supervised placements for nursing students recruited by Project 2000
Diploma in Higher Education programmes introduced after 1986
(National Audit Office, 1992).

This carries important timetabling, as well as ethical, constraints for
continuing educators when arranging practice-based learning experiences, particularly as the priority for learning is usually given to pre-
registration students.

A systematic continuing education programme which carefully avoids a piecemeal approach to teaching and learning is vital according to Kathrein (1990). She argues that effective learning must be sequential, continuous and lifelong, and that to provide anything less than this is to shortchange the learner:

'A pattern of continuing education that comprises intermittent, episodic or discontinuous learning experiences cannot effectively bring about the depth and scope of learning required of professional practitioners. Mere additive experiences (such as reading a journal article followed by an in-service program followed by an external workshop) will not bring about further development unless these experiences relate to and build on one another in an organized pattern of learning based on the individual's learning needs. Discontinuity must be addressed...'

(Kathrein, 1989, p. 216)

The need for purposeful continuity in learning is also stressed by Bysshe (1991) who points to surveys which show that although almost all practitioners in England have had some form of continuing education, much of it is unstructured, uncoordinated and unrecognized:

'There is currently therefore no obvious connection and no frame-work to enable a nurse to progress logically from one level of ability to the next'.

(Bysshe, 1991, p. 19).

However, initiatives from each of the four National Boards for nursing in Britain have since tried to bring order to continuing education by introducing their own systematic 'routes' to higher levels of practice, by inviting practitioners to work towards higher level qualifications.

The problem is that not all service managers perceive the need for continuing education; nor is it necessarily an essential prerequisite for promotion to nurse management posts (Chiarella, 1990).

In a study of continuing professional education for nurses in 1987, Rogers & Lawrence made some 26 recommendations, not the least of which was that all employing health authorities should establish an appropriate relationship between the number of qualified nursing staff, and the number of staff delivering continuing professional education (Rogers & Lawrence, 1987, p. 49). At the very least this would provide employers and policy-makers with some idea of where problems might be realistically tackled.

In setting the future learning agenda, then, our first concern must be for service and education managers to communicate with each other, and to work together to assess both corporate and individual learning needs.

The continuing pace of managerial reform in the NHS and the supremacy of the purchaser-provider ethos in matching service needs with available resources is the prevailing driving force in health care in the early 1990s. Reports from the Audit Commission lend increasing weight to the argument that funding for staff training and development in the past has been distributed haphazardly and unevenly, with no real attempt being made to forecast and target real service demand. The need to recruit and retain staff in line with proper forecasts is also given priority (Audit Commission, 1991, 1992).

Overcoming resistance to demands for new learning

Widespread resistance to the idea of continuing education for staff is less likely if its connection with improved job performance can be established, but this isn't necessarily easy to prove.

The feelings behind such resistance have been explored by several continuing educators and management theorists. Brookfield, for example, says that adults will often be unwilling to expose themselves to their peers, to consider the contextuality of their situations and view their beliefs, behaviours and values as culturally created and therefore provisional (Brookfield, 1986, p. 136).

Because such an activity can be seen as threatening and disturbing, Brookfield says that he can see why teachers might try to withdraw for fear of alienating learners.

He recognizes that teachers of adults find it difficult to strike the right balance, and goes so far as to suggest that there is no point in a teacher rigorously pursuing the critical examination of group members' beliefs if the process is so anxiety-producing that members eventually feel the need to leave the group to restore their self-esteem. Thus, as soon as anxiety becomes a block to learning it has to be rethought from the perspective of the learner. Part of the task of encouraging people to think critically is in helping them to test out their own perceptions in the light of new possibilities.

For example, the ward manager who expresses anger at being asked to develop new skills may feel defensive at first, but given the opportunity to express and discuss his/her fears, may begin to value the opportunities new learning provides to prepare for role-change in the future (Morton-Cooper, 1993).

The fear of being made to look foolish or inadequate in front of colleagues, peers and patients is a very powerful phenomenon, and this is particularly acute in people who have recently returned to practice, changed their job, or conversely, who are established and have worked in the same job for a considerable number of years (Morton-Cooper, 1989).

The need to improve the fit between employees and jobs, learners and learning styles is urgent in health care education, if blocks to learning – and attendant lack of satisfaction in learning and poor uptake of learning opportunities – are to be avoided.

Duplication and repetition of learning already undertaken can also lead to disaffection and withdrawal – a situation which can be avoided with proper assessment of learning and recognition of prior learning and experience.

Blocks to learning need to be handled sensitively, with due regard for the individual, or people will tend to take the easiest route open to them which may be to outwardly conform but inwardly resist (with all the problems this entails); or they may openly resist and become antagonistic and defensive.

In a study which attempts to understand the extent to which different learners experience deterrents or barriers to learning, Valentine & Darkenwald (1990) have gathered together an empirically based typology of adults based on self-reported deterrents to participation, which they describe as 'types' or 'clusters' (see Fig. 1.1).

Although the findings refer to learners in a conventional adult education setting, health professionals constitute a significant number of the adult population and could therefore share many of the same thoughts and feelings.

This typology can be extremely helpful in diagnostic interviews with staff, and serve as a valuable lead-in to discussions about who or what can make continuing professional educational accessible to people with varying professional and personal responsibilities.

Similarly, initiatives to help individuals improve the 'fit' between themselves and their work environment can benefit from straightforward and honest discussion about personal perceptions of learning; the demands and expectations which learning makes on an individual and those closest to them, and most crucial of all, the anticipated outcome of that learning, usually phrased as 'where will this leave me once the course is over?'

Kernoff *et al.* (1989) have produced guidelines for use by nurses in selecting one kind of work environment over another, and this could usefully be adapted for making choices concerning continuing education opportunities.

By combining the identified learning needs of a unit (for example,

Type 1 – People deterred by personal problems (the single largest sub-group, 29.5% of the sample) expressed in the form of family or childcare responsibilities, difficulties with the location, health problems and problems of handicap.

Type 2 – People deterred by lack of confidence (27.2%) The dominant profile here was that of a mature person who lacks the confidence to participate in adult education but who is otherwise in a position to attend.

Type 3 – People deterred by educational costs (the smallest cluster at 12.9% of the sample). Characterized by part-time, predominantly female, employees of 'moderate education and moderate means' who have the confidence to participate but who are unable to afford the direct and indirect costs of learning.

Type 4 – People not interested in organized education (14.3%). Characterized by a well-educated, affluent, working individual, more likely to be male than female, and who places relatively low value on participation in adult education.

Type 5 – People not interested in available courses (16.2%). Disproportionately male group, 83% of whom had college or graduate degrees, classified by the authors as 'highly educated, middle income, working individuals who place considerable value on continuing education but find existing programming irrelevant to their needs'.

Fig. 1.1 A typology of adults based on self-reported deterrents to participation (Valentine & Darkenwald, 1990, p. 36).

intensive care staff who are introducing a new patient transfer scheme) with the personal gaps expressed by the individual, a strategy can be developed which is responsive both to organizational demands, and the self-assessed needs of the staff themselves. (The process of needs assessment is discussed in more detail in Chapter 5.)

Care needs to be taken, however, that we don't effectively disenfranchise learners by giving the impression that 'education' is a process which is most effectively conducted in a college environment. There are times when the reverse may be true. Open and distance learning have had a tremendous impact on the learning culture in nursing education in recent years (see Robinson, 1989).

Also, the suggestion (however subtly transmitted) that education is a process which needs to be superimposed on the workplace, rather than found within it, is a mistake made quite commonly by nurse educators.

Disillusioned with the apparent 'blocks' to learning which confront them in the workplace, (or by the inability to resolve the 'cultural shock' which comes with the 'reality' of nursing work), some nurses attempt to find the answers in the sanctuary of college – Kramer's so-called 'academic lateral arabesquers' (Kramer, 1974, p. 160).

As a consequence, education can become divorced from practice, with both parties vying for dominance in the clinical learning environment. A conflict of values which is unresolved can lead to further dissonance – a situation often described in the literature as the 'theory-practice gap'. Margaret Alexander (1980; 1983) explores this concept and the background to it in depth, as does Kath Melia in her seminal work on the occupational socialization rituals which characterized traditional nurse training prior to the implementation of Project 2000 (Melia, 1987).

Learning 'experientially'

One way in which it is possible to try and close this gap is to recognize the value of personal and shared experience, and to tap their potential for facilitating different kinds of learning. This is a central tenet in the adult education literature, often described as *'experiential learning'*.

One very active proponent of this theme is Burnard (1988). He distinguishes between learning *through* experience (as a situation where an activity is set up through which learning can take place) and learning *from* experience (where students are encouraged to reflect upon past experience as a means of discovering solutions to present problems from past situations (Burnard, 1988, p. 130).

Such a definition echoes the experiential 'learning cycle' put forward by Kolb & Fry (1975, pp. 33–7). Burnard's 'experiential learning cycle for

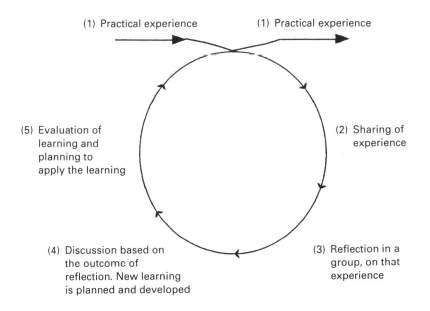

Fig. 1.2 An experiential learning cycle for educational practice (Burnard, 1988, p. 131).

educational practice' whilst not revolutionary (see Fig. 1.2) is an extremely succinct and useful model, capable of wide application in continuing nurse education, and one which can be varied almost indefinitely according to the specific characteristics of learners and the preferred or identified learning needs.

Burnard is sensitive to the fact that tutors or educators are at risk of imposing their own perceptions about situations to learners, and suggests that they act in a facilitating role in the context of experiential learning, allowing learners to explore, question, doubt and criticize their own perceptions, drawing out their own meanings from experience.

Other adult educators who have had a significant impact on continuing nurse education are Rogers (1969; 1980), Gagne (1985), Steinaker & Bell (1979) and Jarvis (1983; 1985).

Rogers' humanistic approach to learning – typified by his assertion that by promoting the concept of 'responsible freedom' in learners it is possible for teachers to be facilitative rather than directive – has been extremely influential in nurse education. His belief that teaching itself is an over-rated activity while learning is under-rated has challenged the beliefs and practices of nurse educators who have been 'syllabus-bound' for many years.

Striking the balance between being skilful in facilitating learning and satisfying the competencies required by qualified nurses has been a difficult nettle for nurse tutors to grasp.

For those who have spent most of their teaching careers in schools of nursing, working in virtual isolation from the clinical area, this difference was originally perceived as an attempt to divest them of their control over teaching, and thus constituted a real threat to their traditional roles as principal players on the nurse education stage.

Rogers' general criticisms of traditional schools' conservatism, rigidity and bureaucracy found fertile ground in British schools and colleges of nursing and midwifery in the 1970s.

His concept of enabling students to *'learn how to learn'*, and the prospects it offered students for empowerment appears to have been slow to take hold, but gradually, as the old-school generation of nurse tutors faded away, their more progressive successors began to respond to the challenge with enthusiasm.

Meanwhile, other forces combined to expose the behaviouristic instructional tendencies of previous educational programmes in nursing which had come about partly for historical and pragmatic reasons, and partly through the work of Gagne whose work was influential in the 1970s.

Gagne (1985) saw value in teachers primarily as instructors and evaluators of students: it was the teachers' job to provide the right 'conditions' for learning, and the students' to respond appropriately to these conditions. For Gagne, then, teacher-centredness and control was the hallmark of education, while for Rogers' it was progression towards student centredness and increasing self-evaluation (Coulter, 1990).

Steinaker & Bell (1979) described an holistic approach to learning, 'an experiential taxonomy', which appeared to fall somewhere in the middle of those ideas presented by Rogers and by Gagne.

This taxonomy takes learners and teachers from an initial *exposure* stage in learning, through that of participation, identification, internalization and dissemination – the last of which enables them to disseminate what they have learned in a critical and analytical way.

This approach is now widely used as a model for curriculum development in both pre- and post-registration education in nursing, and is gaining popularity with Project 2000 designers (see Kenworthy & Nicklin, 1989).

Its potential for clinical teaching is great because it is based on a continuum of immersion in practice from initiation stages to that of dissemination. As such, however, it also carries dangers of returning to covertly behaviouristic (and therefore restrictive) teaching methods and learning outcomes. This is a factor which continuing educators should be alert to when designing learning activities and projects – particularly when planning and negotiating individualized learning. It fits in well with the concept of 'training', and therefore tends to be favoured by employers or educationalists with very specific behavioural outcomes in mind, such as health visiting, occupational health, general practice and health promotion.

Identifying 'teachable moments'

Brookfield's concept of 'teachable moments' is the perfect description for those learning opportunities which present themselves serendipitously. Sadly, they are often overlooked in the rush to structure learning, so that occasions when colleagues could learn from one another in a reciprocal way are not always exploited as much as they could be, given the will and the ability to recognize them.

As Jarvis explains in his book *Professional Education* (1983, p. 83) learning occurs through a variety of interpersonal transactions:

- through self- direction
- facilitation
- being taught
- being instructed
- being trained

- by discussion
- through living
- being socialized
- being influenced
- being conditioned
- being indoctrinated

There are probably others that could be added to this list. What is important in the context of learning support roles is that issues of emotional and learning support are applicable – even fundamental – to each of these transactions in different ways and at different times. The existence of support and the ways in which it is perceived and made available to learners, may be a significant (and previously under-estimated) factor in determining a successful outcome to any learning process; and the reason why elements of support need to be developed and brought into the mainstream of health care education.

In the search for better and more responsive models of teaching in what Krathwohl *et al.* (1964) has described as the *affective domain* of learning (that is, the learning that relates to the feelings, attitudes, emotions and values of the learner), as well as the *cognitive domain* (which involves skills of analysis and recall): increasingly, we will have to recognize both the positive and negative influences which emotional responses can have on a person's willingness and readiness to learn.

Methods for dealing with these aspects of learning can be found in ideas and concepts related to the psychology of stress management; the management of 'transition' and developmental phases in learners' lives and careers; change and adaptation theories; and processes of 'antici-patory socialization' (a means by which people can be prepared for change, and given the support with which they can then be helped to resolve moral conflict and make a positive adaptation).

Reducing stress overload

The damage inflicted by stress is frequently mentioned in the nursing literature – with regard to both staff and their patients. The need to clearly identify occupational stressors and to find appropriate coping strategies is the theme of most writers on this topic (e.g. Hingley & Harris, 1986; Goldenberg & Waddell, 1990; Blake, 1992; McHaffie, 1992).

As McHaffie says, a stressful event can lead to some degree of maturation, if handled well, whereas a less effective coping event may well evoke new conflicts and a reduced state of mental health. She emphasizes that coping 'failures' don't necessarily indicate shortcomings in the individual; rather, the system in which they are placed may have let them down.

Because health workers have a unique opportunity to help people constructively, McHaffie suggests that it is essential that they capitalize on opportunities for their own personal maturation and growth. It is not merely enough to observe specific coping strategies and then to apply knowledge haphazardly:

> 'Systematic research on how people cope in a variety of stressful transactions must go hand in hand with examination of the theory of coping if we are to develop in nursing. Emphasis must be on assisting people to learn to cope with events effectively, both for themselves and their families. Without an understanding of coping, how can a nurse assist families to cope?'
>
> (McHaffie, 1992, p. 939)

In order to reduce unnecessary stress on a ward or similar environment, for example, Simmonds believes that learners must be able to adapt to their new environment and develop interpersonal relationships with regular staff. Failure to do so could otherwise lead them to feel like an 'outsider' (Blake & Simmonds, 1992).

The 'flip' side to this argument, however, is that merely giving people a mechanism for support (such as staff support groups) is to detract from much more important issues (perhaps the environment may be at fault). Is it therefore legitimate or ethical to help staff to try to tolerate the intolerable? As Harvey says: 'Surely the effort should be put into changing the situation rather than changing the people in it?' (Harvey, 1992, p. 257).

Is it worth, therefore, looking closely at the environments and the personalities involved, so that action can be taken to alleviate unnecessary stress and pain? This is a process undertaken very effectively by Pam Smith (1992). By looking at the social construction of 'emotional labour' in nursing, and its subsequent effects on the process of learning, Smith pinpointed the problem with clarity and precision.

Students expressed problems within the dual role of learner and worker, and were incredulous at the lack of support they received through their training from either their teachers or charge nurses:

> 'They felt that there was no one person there for them as an individual. It is little wonder that they talked about becoming cynical in the so-called 'caring profession' that didn't demonstrate any care of its most junior and largest group of carers'
>
> (Smith, 1992, p. 128)

Smith concluded that while nursing leaders exhorted nurses to care, their definitions of caring were too limited to take the emotional complexity of caring into account, even though caring was considered to be an essential ingredient of 'good nursing':

> 'Student nurses felt better able to care for patients when they felt cared for themselves by the trained ward staff and their teachers ... The accounts of caring from both students and patients suggested that 'caring' does not come naturally. Nurses have to work emotionally on themselves in order to appear to care, irrespective of how they personally feel about themselves, individual patients, their conditions and circumstances'

(Smith, 1992, p. 128)

However, Smith also suggested that it was possible for nurses (and presumably their colleagues) to be *taught* how to manage their feelings more effectively. This brings us back to the demand for a sensitive approach from employers and educators as in the different stages and transitions we go through during our personal and work-related development.

It is also argued that part of becoming reflective practitioners is the need to respond with insight to anxiety-related and avoidance behaviours; to confront fears and to actively deal with them in a manner compatible with our values.

The appropriate use of role models which will 'give permission' for the admission of difficult experiences is one important way in which support can be made accessible to learners, whatever their chronological or maturational stage of development (Newell, 1992).

In essence, that is exactly what this book is about. In the pages that follow, we will be exploring the possibilities for greater use of support roles, and, in particular, those of mentorship and preceptorship.

Rigid demarcations about where one role begins and another ends has dogged the effective use of such roles in British health care education, and perhaps blinded us to their much wider potential. The reasons for this are discussed in the chapters which follow.

The education of equals

Finally, as Jarvis warns, it is important for nurses to recognize that a dominant model in the practice of education is apparent in the UK, a model he describes as 'education from above' (such as the majority of examination syllabi in initial education, and probably also in professional education). He argues that the continuation of such a model can only be justified if it is successful in occupational terms (Jarvis, 1986, p. 467).

Given the wealth of evidence bearing witness to its flaws, traditional nurse training could not easily be said to be successful for all sorts of reasons (e.g. Commission on Nursing Education, RCN, 1985), hence the emergence of Project 2000 and the current radical reform of British nursing education (UKCC, 1986; 1991).

The major question now is whether, as Jarvis says, nursing requires practitioners who are compliant to the demands from above, or whether it needs those who are able to be self-directing?

Jarvis also infers that despite the suspicion that developing on the premise of 'education as equals' could lead to management and containment problems in the service, ('notions of mutiny and insurrection?'), it is possible to legislate for this by providing senior staff with a knowledge and understanding of the educational process. His argument appears to be based on the premise that those who are made aware of the nature of the educational process are more likely to emphasize with it, plan for it, lead it, *and* make it happen.

The promise of 'education as equals' rather than 'education from above' then is central to the thesis of learning support. More importantly, the ways in which we can help to make it happen are considered next, when we demonstrate the evolution and application of support roles to health care practice.

References

Alexander, M. (1980) *Nurse Education: An Experiment in Integration of Theory and Practice in Nursing.* PhD thesis, University of Edinburgh.

Alexander, M. (1983) *Learning to Nurse – Integrating Theory and Practice.* Churchill Livingstone, Edinburgh.

Audit Commission (1991) *The Virtue of Patients: Making Best Use of Ward Nursing Resources.* HMSO, London.

Audit Commission (1992) *Making Time for Patients: A Handbook for Ward Sisters.* HMSO, London.

Best, F. & Stern, B. (1976) *Lifetime Distribution of Education, Work and Leisure.* Institute for Educational Leadership, Post Secondary Convening Authority, Washington DC.

Blake, R. & Simmonds, J. (1992) Stress levels in nurse education. *Senior Nurse,* **12**, 3, 16–17.

Boud, D. (ed) (1981) *Developing Student Autonomy in Learning.* Kogan Page, London.

Boud, D., Keogh, R. & Walker, M. (1985) *Reflection: Turning Experience into Learning*. Kogan Page, London.

Bradby, M.B. (1990) Status Passage into Nursing: Undertaking Nursing Care. *Journal of Advanced Nursing*, **15**, 1363–9.

Brookfield, S.D. (1986) *Understanding and Facilitating Adult Learning*. Open University Press, Milton Keynes.

Brookfield, S.D. (1987) *Developing Critical Thinkers – Challenging Adults to Explore New Ways of Thinking and Acting*. Open University Press, Milton Keynes.

Burnard, P. (1988) Experiential learning: some theoretical considerations. *International Journal of Lifelong Education*, **7**, 2, 127–33.

Bysshe, J. (1991) PREPP and TNA: Where's the Catch? *Nursing*, **4**, 32, 18–21.

Cervero, R.M. (1992) Professional practice, learning and continuing education: an integrated perspective, *International Journal of Lifelong Education*, **11**, 2, 91–101.

Chiarella, E.M. (1990) Developing the credibility of continuing education. *Nurse Education Today*, **2**, 70–73.

Coulter, M.A. (1990) A review of two theories of learning and their application in the practice of nurse education. *Nurse Education Today*, **10**, 333–8.

Cross, K.P. (1981) *Adults as Learners*. Jossey Bass, San Francisco.

Curtis, S.J. & Boultwood, M. (1964) *An Introductory History of English Education*. Tutorial Press Limited, University of London.

Davenport, J. (1993) Is there any way out of the andragogy morass? in Thorpe, M., Edwards, R., Hanson, A. (eds) *Culture and Processes of Adult Learning*, pp. 109–117. Routledge/The Open University.

Dearden, R.F. (1990) in Esland, G. (ed) *Education, Training and Employment*, pp. 84–95. The Open University/Addison Wesley, Milton Keynes and London.

Dewey, J. (1933) *How We Think*. Heath Publishers, New York.

Downie, R.S. & Charlton, B. (1992) *The Making of a Doctor – Medical Education in Theory and Practice*. Oxford University Press, Oxford.

Freire, P. (1972) *Pedagogy of the Oppressed*. Penguin, Harmondsworth.

Gagne, R.M. (1985) (3rd edition) *The Conditions of Learning*. Holt, Rinehart and Winston, New York.

Glen, S. (1990) Power for nursing education. *Journal of Advanced Nursing*, **15**, 1335–40.

Goldenberg, D. & Waddell, J. (1990) Occupational stress and coping strategies among female baccalaureate nursing faculty. *Journal of Advanced Nursing*, **15**, 531–43.

Harvey, P. (1992) Staff support groups: are they necessary? *British Journal of Nursing*, **1**, 5, 256–8.

Hingley, P. & Harris, P. (1986) Lowering the tension. *Nursing Times*, **82**, 32, 52–3.

Jarvis, P. (1983) *Professional Education*. Croom Helm, London.

Jarvis, P. (1985) *The Sociology of Adult and Continuing Education*. Croom Helm, London.

Jarvis, P. (1986) Nurse education and adult education: a question of the person. *Journal of Advanced Nursing*, **11**, 465–9.

Jowett, B. (trans) (1899) *The Politics of Aristotle*. Colonial Press, New York.

Kathrein, M.A. (1990) Continuing nursing education: a perspective. *The Journal of Continuing Education in Nursing*, **21**, 5, 216– 18.

Kenworthy, N. & Nicklin, P. (1989) *Teaching and Assessing in Nursing Practice – An Experiential Approach*. Scutari Press, London.

Kernoff, P. Yu, L., McCool, W. & Packard, J.S. (1989) The job context index: a guide for improving the 'fit' between nurses and their work environment. *Journal of Advanced Nursing*, **14**, 501–8.

Knowles, M.S. (1980) *The Modern Practice of Adult Education: From Pedagogy to Andragogy*. (2nd ed) Cambridge Books, New York.

Knowles, M.S. (1984) *Andragogy in Action – Applying Modern Principles of Adult Learning*. Jossey Bass, San Francisco.

Kolb, D.A. & Fry, R. (1975) Towards an applied theory of experiential learning, in Cooper, C.L. (ed) *Theories of Group Processes* John Wiley & Sons, London

Kramer, M. (1974) Postgraduation nurse socialization: an emergent theory, in *Reality Shock: Why Nurses Leave Nursing*, CV Mosby & Co, St Louis.

Krathwohl, D.R., Bloom, B.S., Masia, B.B. (1964) *Taxonomy of Educational Objectives: The Classification of Educational Goals, Handbook II, Affective Domain*. David McKay, New York.

Leddy, S. & Pepper, J.M. (1989) *Conceptual Bases of Professional Nursing* (2nd ed). Lippincott & Co, Philadelphia.

Marsick, V.J. (ed) (1987) New Paradigms for Learning in the Workplace, in *Learning in the Workplace*, pp. 11–30. Croom Helm, London.

McHaffie, H.E. 1992) Coping: an essential element in nursing, *Journal of Advanced Nursing*, **17**, 933–40.

Melia, K.M. (1987) *Learning and Working: the Occupational Socialisation of Nurses*. Churchill Livingstone, Edinburgh.

Mezirow, J. (1983) A critical theory of adult learning and education, in Tight, M. (ed) *Adult Learning and Education*, Vol. 1. Croom Helm/The Open University, Beckenham and Milton Keynes.

Mezirow, J. (ed) (1990) *Fostering Critical Reflection in Adulthood – A Guide to Transformative and Emancipatory Learning*. Jossey Bass, San Francisco.

Morton-Cooper, A. (1989) *Returning to Nursing – A Guide for Nurses and Health Visitors*. Macmillan, Basingstoke.

Morton-Cooper, A. (1993) 'Educating for Role Change'. Management Education Conference, *Journal of Nursing Management*/Dudley Road Hospital, Birmingham, 21 September.

National Audit Office (1992) *Nursing Education: Implementation of Project 2000 in England*. HMSO, London.

Newell, R. (1992) Anxiety, accuracy and reflection: the limits of professional development. *Journal of Advanced Nursing*, **17**, 1326–33.

Nutton, V. (1992) Healers in the medical marketplace: towards a social history of Graeco-Roman medicine, in Wear, A. (ed) *Medicine in Society – Historical Essays*. Cambridge University Press, Cambridge.

Ozman, H. & Raven, S. (1990) (4th edition) *Philosophical Foundations of Education.* C.E. Merrill Publishing Co., Columbus, Ohio.

Pietroni, P. (1991) *The Greening of Medicine.* Victor Gollancz, London.

RCN (1985) *The Education of Nurses: a New Dispensation.* (the Judge Commission), Royal College of Nursing, London.

Riegelman, R.K., Povar, G.J., Ott, J.E. & Piemme, T.E. (1985) A strategy for the education of 21st century physicians, *Medical Teacher*, **7**, 3/4, 279–83.

Robinson, K. (ed) (1989) *Open and Distance Learning for Nurses.* Longman Group, Harlow, Essex.

Rogers, C.R. (1969) *Freedom to Learn.* C.E. Merrill Publishing Co, Columbus, Ohio.

Rogers, C.R. (1980) *Freedom to Learn for the Eighties.* C.E. Merrill Publishing Co, Columbus, Ohio.

Rogers, J. & Lawrence, J. (1987) *Continuing Professional Education for Qualified Nurses, Midwives and Health Visitors.* Institute of Education, University of London, London.

Salvage, J. (1986) *The Politics of Nursing.* Heinemann, London.

Schon, D. (1983) *The Reflective Practitioner: How Professionals Think in Action.* Basic Books, New York.

Seivwright, M.J. (1988) How to develop tomorrow's nursing leaders. *International Nursing Review*, **35**, 4, 99–106.

Silcock, P. (1991) Learning nursing: what factors are responsible for a lack of creativity. *Nursing Practice*, **4**, 3, 24–8.

Simmonds, J. & Blake, R. (1992) Stress levels in nurse education, *Senior Nurse*, **12**, 3, 16–19.

Smith, P. (1992) *The Emotional Labour of Nursing.* Macmillan, Basingstoke.

Steinaker, N.W. & Bell, M.R. (1979) *The Experiential Taxonomy.* Academic Press, New York.

Tennant, M. (1988) *Psychology and Adult Learning*, Routledge, London.

Toffler, A. (1970) *Future Shock.* Random House, New York.

Townsend, P., Davidson, N. & Whitehead, M. (1988) *Inequalities in Health.* Penguin Books, London.

UKCC (1986) *Project 2000 – A New Preparation for Practice.* UKCC, London.

UKCC (1990) *The Report of the Post-Registration Education and Practice Project* (PREPP report), UKCC, London.

Valentine, T. & Darkenwald, G.G. (1990) Deterrents to participation in adult education: profiles of the potential learners, *Adult Education Quarterly*, **41**, 1, 29–42.

World Health Organization (WHO) (1979) *Formulating Strategies for Health for All*, WHO, Geneva.

Chapter 2
Introduction to Support Roles

Why support systems are needed

Support systems of a sort have always existed in health care, whether they have come about naturally or informally, as friendships, shared confidences between peers, as part of organized educational activities or the more formal quasi-counselling which happens between managers and their staff.

So why should we, the authors, consider setting up a more formal structure which may well lead to more expense, more administration and the possibility of more valuable time being deflected away from patient care?

The changing working culture

The current focus is that of a learning culture to assist individuals, organizations and society to collectively come to terms with, and benefit from, the rapid technological changes now taking place. We need to be able to make use of the finite resources that are available, and to come to an understanding about what it means to live and work in what is being identified as the post-Fordist society (Hogget, 1987; Murray, 1991). Post-Fordism relates to the postmodernist changes currently occurring in society, bought about by advances in technology, modern communication and information systems. Whether it is part of a general social trend (Harvey, 1990), or a cultural transformation of some significance (Wilkin, 1993), remains to be seen.

Fordism was characterized by mass manufacturing production techniques (for example, Henry Ford and the car industry), factories, and goods and services for the masses (Edwards, 1991). This resulted in organizational cultures and institutions that were mainly authoritarian and hierarchical; large bureaucracies maintained and controlled by central planning and restrictive practices (Edwards, 1991). This has begun to change with the shift of emphasis to post-Fordism, where the main principles are flexibility, targeting specific markets, and quality assurance. There has been a move away from the solid manufacturing base of the industrial revolution towards the provision of convenience goods and 'softer' service industries, to the offices, shops, leisure centres and fast food facilities. There are those who argue that the post-Fordist future will result in a very different social formation:

- '25% will be skilled workers with permanent jobs in large firms protected by collective wage agreements;
- 25% will be peripheral workers with insecure, unskilled and badly paid jobs, whose work schedules vary according to the wishes of their employers and the fluctuations in the market;
- 50% will be semiemployed, unemployed, or marginalized workers, doing occasional or seasonal work of odd jobs'.   (Gorz, 1989)

A post-Fordist society is one where rapid change is inevitable, competition for resources high and where personal work patterns and consumer expectations will be vastly different from those of previous generations.

In response to the changes, a variety of nations have identified their priorities and strategies for better informed societies by devising projects or legislation that has led to initiatives for greater participation in higher education. In the UK there is a recognized need to keep pace with what is happening and to implement policies for economic growth that will affect productivity and increase consumer confidence (Ball, 1992). The resulting change to that of the competitive internal market is currently being felt within a diverse range of established British public services – notably transport, education and health.

The changing UK health service

Health care is becoming increasingly more complex. Recent policy changes in the UK (DoH, 1989) have resulted in the creation of a managed market with emphasis on business strategies and purchaser/provider roles. Control and management of health services has been relocated to District Health Authorities (DHAs), and a more streamlined National Health Service (NHS) now exists with clearly identified executive and general management functions. There has been a shift in emphasis from consensus management of the early 1980s to general management functions for the 1990s. The principles of efficiency, effectiveness and value for money underpin the drive for a market approach to health care. Those working in the service and those being treated are steadily coming to terms with self-governing trusts and the purchasing, providing and contracting principles of health care.

Currently a bilateral system exists with some hospitals and communities remaining within the remit of the NHS, now known as Directly Managed Units, and others having 'opted out' and become Hospital and Community Trusts. Both are in direct competition to provide services for the DHAs. The Trusts appear as self-governing institutions with clinical directorates that demonstrate a clear business approach to the organization of health services. New structures, missions and languages are becoming apparent as the DHAs form different working relationships and come to terms with their new purchaser/provider roles within the rigours of an internal market for health. The new relationships that appear to be forming are illustrated in diagrammatic form in Fig. 2.1. Within this changing model of health care provision, general practitioners in the community are allocated their own budgets and can purchase care for their patients and clients from the choice of providers available.

The demands in the form of new technology, the rapid turnover of patients/clients, alternative models of education and health, and newly proposed community initiatives, are ever increasing. The patient as a consumer has rising expectations, and the newly introduced concept by the Government of 'citizen's rights' has added to the burdens being placed upon practitioners (DoH, 1992). The implications of rapid change and increasing challenges have begun to test even the most experienced of health care practitioners in recent years. Many health service staff feel they are being carried along on an unstoppable tide of change and confusion (George, 1986).

It is important at such a time of challenge and turbulence to make the most of the available human resources, and to tap into their valuable potential. It would also appear to be a sensible option to draw on the available, relevant theoretical principles of individual potential and motivation to provide supportive frameworks that are enabling and flexible in order to meet the needs and requirements of both the individuals and the organization. It is also vital to consider supportive relationships, whereby care workers and professional practitioners can feel free to develop at their own rate and in their own terms. This can be achieved by devising a range of support mechanisms that encourages individual growth and personal development by offering caring assistance that, in turn, facilitates the sharing of relevant expertize and appropriate standards of care. Such supportive frameworks will enhance motivation, encourage creativity, stimulate risk-taking, nurture developing leadership qualities, and benefit patient care.

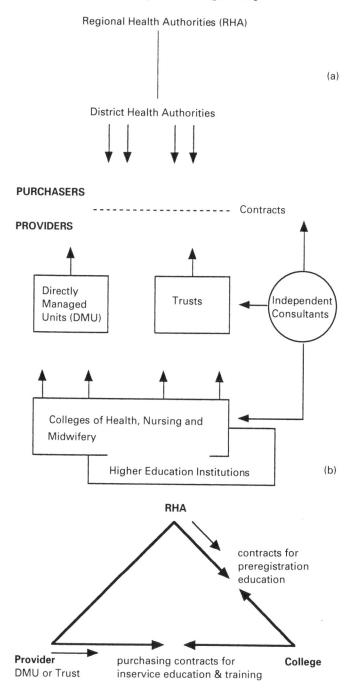

Fig. 2.1 New relationships in the health service. (a) Purchaser-provider relationships; (b) emerging model of nurse education contracting relationships.

The challenge is to take the initiative and prepare an effective case for strengthening existing support frameworks, and to develop new ones as part of the ongoing debate concerning staff development and the need for continuing professional education. The route will not be an easy one: the essentials of value-for-money, cost-effectiveness, and 'proof of worth' have rapidly gained ground. The continuing demise of the NHS and arrival of Trust status with the notion of independence and an ethos of purchasing and providing has led to a new and volatile ingredient in the UK health service – that of internal competition. It remains vitally important at such a time that new ideas and the sharing of good practice across districts continues.

There are increasing signs that the newly formed Trusts' search for value-for-money will place a greater emphasis on the functional needs of the organization as a whole. This may be to the detriment of the personal learning and support needs of those working in the service. Sound arguments will have to be used to convince the purchasers and providers that establishing formal support frameworks will benefit both practitioners and the patients in their care. This will have to be achieved at a time of increased cost implications and when there is increased competition for the limited finances that are available.

The case for support systems

In this era of rapid change and reorientation to new thinking and acting, people have a natural tendency to feel uncertain. As Broome (1990) explains, it is the balance of the individual's internal state and skill, and the support and encouragement that he or she receives from the surroundings that will determine the capacity to deal with uncertainty:

> 'If individuals are put under too much pressure they will resist change, but if they are part of an organization that values change, then they are more likely to take risks and to contribute more to the change effect.'
>
> Broome (1990, p. 48).

Broome stresses the need to look at the *total environment in which we expect people to function* in order to join in the change process and perform to their greatest potential. This includes an assessment of the demands of the everyday work situation, in balance with the private and personal responsibilities and the stressors individuals bring with them.

All this will affect the capacity to take on new ideas, new behaviours and new practices. On one day a person's capacity may be greater than on another due to a wide range of restraining factors. An efficient manager will be in touch with these factors, note the individual's capacity to take on new challenges at different times and will match the change process accordingly (Broome, 1990, p. 48).

Support is about being sensitive to the human dynamics that surround us. It is also about allowing individuals to be self-directive and assisting them to manage the change process for themselves. By providing a workable 'helping' relationship we can start to communicate properly, build effective partnerships and get beyond some of the limiting attitudes and behaviours which make up a negative hierarchy at work. Such helping relationships can also assist in addressing the concerns about burnout and diminished staff morale, common to those in helping professions which result in a range of avoiding behaviours and high absenteeism, (Daley, 1979).

Learning support

Supportive helping relationships assist individuals to plan their development by:

- Working out individual learning requirements.
- Formulating career outcomes.
- Evaluating own role and performance within the organization.
- Building self concept in career socialisation terms.

Appropriate support can aid development by providing an ongoing, interactive dialogue whereby individuals can contemplate moving from accepting concrete, factual knowledge to demonstrating their abilities to deal with and solve complex problems as part of their continuing professional education.

Taking responsibility for their own learning involves placing a value on past experiences and being able to relate these experiences to current practice. Supportive relationships assist this process of self-discovery, helping individual practitioners to clarify their personal and career needs in order to discover their own personal style; and this is then demonstrated in their practice. To make this more meaningful there is a need to integrate past experiences, and to learn through experience (Kolb, 1984; Weil & McGill, 1989). For the professional practitioner the processes are those of 'learning through'. This entails the thinking about doing, the actual doing, the thinking through doing and the thinking about what was done and is still to be done. Appropriate support frameworks can provide individuals with personal 'time out' for reflection in and on action, as suggested by Schon (1987).

In an increasingly complex world where there are few set patterns for practice or concrete answers, preparing practitioners via the skills of their own reflections appears a sensible and viable option. It challenges our views on what constitutes learning. This is explained well by Barnett (1990) who calls for insight, involvement and reflection ... not learning as such:

> 'Students have to show that they understand what has been learned so deeply that they are able to look down on it and assess it critically for themselves.'

> (Barnett, 1990, p. 151)

To assist these processes and encourage critical reflection, clearly identifiable frameworks are required to make the best use of available experienced practitioners in a variety of support roles. The roles contained within such frameworks extend beyond those formed as friendships, peers, role models, facilitators or supervisors.

Emotional support

Egan's model of the skilled helper is a telling one for health care professionals because it is based on concepts of pragmatism (the real world), competence (problem-solving), respect (non-judgemental), and genuineness (spontaneity, non-defensiveness, consistency and openness), (Egan, 1990, p. 56).

Responsiveness to individual concerns and to helping employees find new ways of dealing with stress and uncertainty is a complex part of management and leadership functions.

It is often argued that emotions are signals that accompany the transitions between one kind of action and another. Emotions are alarm bells, indicating that something important has occurred. With an emotion, we become ready to continue what we were doing or respond by doing something else (Oatley & Johnson Laird, 1987). When our role is under threat or lost, then the emotions become the mechanism through which we manage the transition from one phase to another: they either sustain us or they don't.

It would seem reasonable to assume therefore that support through an emotional phase or given an ability to understand where our emotions can lead us can be a very powerful force for helping us to move forward personally, socially and professionally.

Marquis & Huston (1992) have identified ten 'emotional phases' which are passed through as part of the change process (see Table 2.1). The potential for support roles in helping staff to feel part of the inevitable change process rather than as a passive bystander is therefore enormous. Changing work roles, patterns and structures in health care requires everyone to take the management of change seriously. The introduction of support systems to help us to cope and manage change is therefore vital if we are to survive the challenges that lie ahead.

General support and development framework

With the current complexities and demands for health care it would appear a sensible option to provide a support framework that is designed to meet the changing requirements of professional practice. Such frameworks should be flexible and comprehensive to include the many differing development phases, and transition periods in a professional practitioner's career. It should be a framework designed specifically to draw together the range of support and development roles that are now available, in order to assist those engaged in the increasing rigours of professional practice. It is important to note that such a framework

Table 2.1   Ten emotional phases of the change process.

1.	**Equilibrium**	Characterized by high energy, and emotional and intellectual balance. Personal and professional goals are synchronized.
2.	**Denial**	Individual denies reality of the change. Negative changes occur in physical, cognitive and emotional functioning.
3.	**Anger**	Energy is manifested by rage, envy and resentment.
4.	**Bargaining**	In an attempt to eliminate the change, energy is expended by bargaining.
5.	**Chaos**	Characterized by diffused energy, feelings of powerlessness, insecurity, and loss of identity.
6.	**Depression**	Defence mechanisms are no longer operable. No energy left to produce results. Self-pity apparent.
7	**Resignation**	Change accepted passively but without enthusiasm.
8	**Openness**	Some renewal of energy in implementing new roles or assignments that have resulted from the change.
9	**Readiness**	Wilful expenditure of energy to explore new event. Physical, cognitive and emotional reunification occurs.
10.	**Re-emergence**	Individual again feels empowered and begins initiating projects and ideas.

(*Source*: Marquis & Huston, 1992, from *Leadership Roles and Management Functions in Nursing – Theory and Applications*. J.B. Lippincott).

should not be entirely created to respond to need alone as this may cause imbalances for some, and may result in increased responses to demand from others (Earwaker, 1992).

What is required are well-defined initiatives and a clear strategy that will provide a supportive network of support-orientated individuals. These individuals should be capable and prepared to work together, to take on the many different roles that are now available.

A more well-defined interpretation and enhanced understanding of the roles and functions available may aid in breaking down the prejudices – particularly of those sceptical to the use of mentoring as it is currently being 'used' in clinical practice. The language employed to describe mentoring in the recent past concerning that of protégés and distortions towards sponsorship elements has led to associations with elitism and favouritism which may not rest well within the public service sector. Mentoring and preceptorship, if understood and applied appropriately, provide such support systems by complementing and adding to the value of the roles already available.

The concepts of mentoring and preceptorship are fully examined in Chapters 3 and 4. Our intention here is to present an overview of the possible available support mechanisms for a variety of settings. The main elements of a proposed supportive framework form the discussion for the remainder of this chapter. Although intended primarily for nurses, midwives and health visitors in this instance, it could well be adapted to provide a framework of support for others involved in health care where similar professional entrances and routes exist.

A broader notion of support than has necessarily been considered in the past is envisaged: supportive frameworks are needed to form part of the wider remit of staff development to aid those starting out, as well as those actively engaged in professional practice, assisting them to cope with the new challenges and increasing tensions. We suggest that the basis for such a comprehensive framework can be categorized into four main areas of support requirement. These relate to the individual's learning and developmental needs in terms of his/her point of entry and specific changes in professional circumstances. These are the four areas selected and identified in the framework:

(1) Entry to the profession – *the student.*
(2) Entry as a professional practitioner – *newly qualified.*
(3) Transition periods of re-entry and role change – *the qualified.*
(4) Moving to influence the profession – *qualified and experienced.*

The support framework as presented matches the key roles judged to be the most applicable for the stage of development or transition event that is occurring. This match is based upon current available research, our experiences in practice and education, and with regard to inter-pretations of nursing, midwifery and health visiting guidelines (UKCC, 1993).

The ideas for the framework can be represented in diagrammatic form as shown in Fig. 2.2 – a general support and development framework. This identifies the areas and individuals for support and incorporates the significant roles and relationships, linking them to produce a vital matrix of support. This establishes a social network of practitioners, defined as the collective title for the individuals and organizational systems with which there is communication (Barker, 1990).

Support for the student is demonstrated in the recognizable roles of group colleagues, educational support and a proposed, new clinical role, that of the *facilitator-coach*. This role will be explored in more detail later in the chapter.

Preceptor support is identified for qualified staff who are engaged in some form of role transition. The qualified, experienced practitioner may alternatively be offered access to formal support by way of a con-tract or formal mentor, as part of a formal mentoring programme. These programmes could be offered for qualified staff as part of a recognized staff development strategy. A contract mentor, by providing an essen-tially collaborative relationship of personal equality, could help develop those experienced, qualified staff who wished to take more responsi-bility to:

● Develop effective leadership qualities.
● Broaden their professional network.
● Begin to influence the profession.

Naturally chosen, career relationships such as those of classical men-toring should be allowed to develop spontaneously. Relationships are fluid, flexible and dynamic. Some specified functional roles such as preceptorship may extend beyond their identified 'shelf life', given the right mix of personal qualities, enough time and the relevant contact to develop mutual trust, respect and the enabling intimacy of classical mentoring. The classical mentor is included in Fig. 2.2 to show how it can be available to all personnel in the organization, and fit into the general scheme of supportive relationships.

Support and development for the student

The particular needs of qualified staff are covered in Chapters 3 and 4 in relation to the nature, functions and responsibilities of mentors and

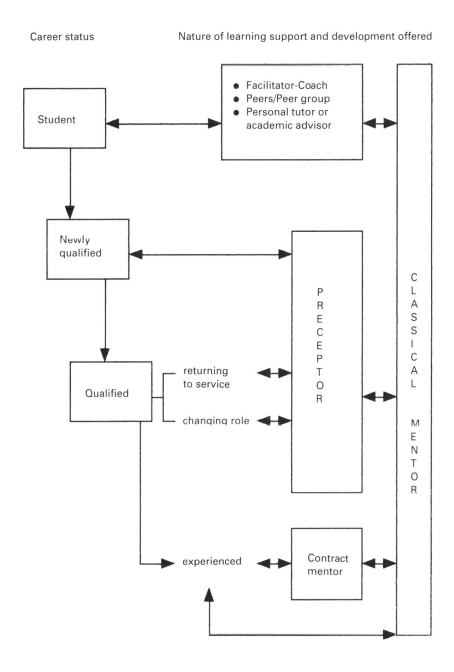

Fig. 2.2 General support framework incorporating significant roles and relationships.

preceptors. It is the intention at this point to confine discussions to the aspects of the support framework that relate particularly to the student – who, as a new arrival, has particular educational, clinical learning and support needs. The discussion will highlight some familiar support roles in the form of peers and tutorial advisers as well as introduce different, modified roles in the form of a broader interpretation for that of the previously identified clinical supervisor.

Student support is complemented by a wider network of significant others in the form of their peers and educational advisers who may be designated as personal tutors or academic advisers. Such roles are identified in relation to student needs, but it is worth noting at this juncture that any qualified practitioner who registers for a further course of study will have access to these others. In the support framework the role of facilitator-coach is identified primarily for the student at the point of entry to the profession.

Peers and peer groups

A peer is a colleague who is of similar status within the organization; someone who forms a collaborative relationship that is often mutually rewarding. The relationship is also non-competitive in nature. The peer group consists of a collection of peers which forms an informal and supportive social network where the individuals relate together as colleagues and friends.

As discussed earlier in this chapter, health care is becoming more complicated and change more rapid, making the demands for care provision more exacting. Similar demands are now occurring in education. Changes in the student population, with the numbers of mature students gradually increasing, and living patterns changing have meant fewer opportunities for the formal and informal exchanges. These were characterized by the shared practices that arose from close working relationships in clinical placements and by the informal opportunities for reflection on practical experiences arising from living in communal establishments within close proximity to the patients.

Peers and peer groups can provide the student with a close, social network that can be very beneficial to the student, allowing him/her to gain a great deal from this type of liaison. Remaining as part of the group can assist the student in checking personal progress within the relative safety of a group of colleagues of similar standing. The desire to make use of the potential benefits of this sort of grouping has led to the setting up of more formal systems of peer groups; peer tutorials, The Open University, self-help groups, the *Nursing Times* Open Learning student study groups and the Buddy systems of North America are helpful examples. All these systems offer a variety of different approaches to assist students to become part of their own independently directed groups, and lead to increasing initiatives for student contribution to peer review, peer audit, peer evaluation and co-counselling (Burnard, 1988; Kenworthy & Nicklin, 1989).

The roles and responsibilities of academic advisers

Academic advisers have a central role to play in supporting students through an education programme. They are assigned to students to assist with their progress on the course. They do this by helping the student to set his/her own realistic academic goals or targets which can then be achieved. The student is encouraged to be self-directed and to make the most of the learning opportunities that occur during and outside the timetabled sessions of the curriculum.

The academic adviser is usually a member of the course team and this knowledge of the course programme and commitments eases the student through the rigours of academic life. This has become an increasingly important priority as new educational initiatives are placed on the educational agenda. Initiatives of accreditation of prior learning, and accreditation of prior experiential learning have resulted in increasing numbers of mature students with different abilities. This is providing educational managers, lecturers and advisors with the challenges of managing the increasing numbers and discovering new methods and approaches of encouraging learning (Ramsden, 1992).

Choosing the right course, working through modules, as well as pressures of continuing assessment and self-direction, make it appropriate for the student to have a significant academic helper. Changing social circumstances and taking increasing responsibility for learning and progression through a course may increase risks of student isolation. Students are obliged to know who to contact in order to ensure that their academic needs will be met (Rickards, 1992).

The responsibility for arranging meetings and tutorials rest with the student who is encouraged to meet regularly in order for the academic adviser to assist in assessing progress and in helping the student to reach his/her full academic potential. The specific roles and functions of the academic adviser are itemized below and demonstrate the range of responsibilities that play a major part in the student's academic development.

For the individual student, the responsibilities of the academic adviser are:

To help:

- make the most effective use of time,
- to plan an individual programme of work,
- set realistic targets,
- choose the options that best meet personal needs, interests and career plans,
- in liaising with the teaching staff or registry.

To reflect:

- on individual development in relation to the course, and to chart progress.

To monitor:

- progress on the course in light of the personal and academic goals set.

To provide:

- advice and career references that may be required in the future.

(University of London, The Centre for Higher Educational Studies, 1992)

In this manner the student is given support that reflects his/her individual learning needs during the course. The academic support and assistance relates to all aspects of the course to include help with organizational aspects, such as administration, and extends beyond the end of the course to that of the working world.

Personal tutors

Another common support role with responsibilities similar to those of the academic adviser is that of the personal tutor. As a member of the teaching staff, the personal tutor is important, providing the student with support and having 'responsibilities for keeping a watchful eye on the student's work and progress on an individual basis' (Earwaker, 1992, pp. 45–6).

Traditionally in nursing education, medicine and other health care programmes, the personal tutor has had responsibilities that extended beyond those of the academic adviser (Taylor, 1980). As well as assisting with the student's academic progress, the personal tutor had responsibilities for pastoral care and overseeing the student's progress through practice placements. Prior to the advent of Project 2000 courses (UKCC, 1986) and the change of student status to that of supernumerary, the personal tutor's counselling role did not always fit easily with the management responsibilities of 'the employed student'. Recognizing this, counselling services were developed in some nursing schools but in the main, student counselling responsibilities remained with the personal tutor. In higher education, pastoral support is available from a variety of institutional sources such as student services and specialized telephone help-lines. The academic adviser can therefore concentrate on helping the student to reach his/her academic potential and make appropriate counselling referrals should the need arise. The clear distinction in responsibilities is made and the personal tutor's role is to assist the student to set his/her own learning agenda 'within a business-like working relationship' (Earwaker, 1992).

Setting the scene: supervision and facilitation

A variety of key roles have previously been identified in providing learning support for students in clinical placements. These have been instrumental in developing those new to the professional working world. In social work and occupational therapy, clinical supervisors have responsibilities for assisting learning and clinical socialization. In midwifery, health visiting and nursing, the roles of clinical supervisors, field-work practice teachers, clinical teachers, assessors and, latterly, mentors have been established to enhance learning and provide learning support. The emphasis in the past has been on the use of clinical supervision to prepare students and to provide role models for practice.

Supervision

Supervision in areas of general nursing has become too specifically focused on mainly punitive, monitoring elements. Ogier & Cameron Buccheri (1990) report the dissatisfaction with supervision of the past in nursing but suggest that:

> 'Supportive, competent supervision is essential if nurses are to give their best to the care of the ill, frail and vulnerable.'

> (Ogier & Cameron Buccheri, 1990, p. 24)

As a result of the past difficulties associated with supervision, new roles were formulated, particularly for student groups, as curriculum planning was under way during the early stages of Project 2000 implementation. This comprehensive and far-reaching report was the nursing profession's response to the challenge of providing effective nursing care into the next century. Concerns regarding changes in primary care and the rise in the number of elderly patients, required a nursing work force adequately prepared and competent to deliver a high standard of care. The main proposals were:

- Integration of nursing education and higher education.
- Implementation of student status.
- Reform of preregistration courses.
- A single grade of nurse.

This resulted in raising the level of debate on issues of skill-mix, enrolled nurse conversion, nursing college amalgamations, and the identification of a new and different clinical support role – that of the mentor. To assist in the development of the 'knowledgeable doer', this interpretation of the mentor role involved supervisory and assessment activities.

Barber & Norman (1987) suggest that supervisory relationships can be viewed more positively in other areas, such as social work and mental health. Here, supervision is more widely interpreted as being open and enabling, drawing on psychotherapy and counselling techniques to provide an openly facilitative relationship for those concerned.

In suggesting that the supervisor of midwives role should be developed, the UKCC (1991) recognized the role as that of a supportive colleague, counsellor and adviser to other midwives with the aim of maintaining and improving practice; a sound suggestion if the supervisor:midwife ratios are realistically determined to support the enabling aspects expected of such relationships. Barber & Norman (1987) consider that others could learn from a wider interpretation of clinical supervision and the recent text by Butterworth & Faugier (1992) supports this view.

A comprehensive case is made for revisiting supervision in its broadest sense, to benefit both the practitioners and those they care for. Professional supervision of this nature involves setting ground rules for practice and the use of effective information (Johns, 1993). The supervisory relationship is seen as one that is both collaborative and collegial in assisting supervised individuals to learn through, and from, their experiences to aid personal development and effectiveness.

Facilitation

In interpreting a broader, more fitting role for the current climate if supervisory elements remain unacceptable, it is suggested that facilitation be considered. The art of facilitation has been well-documented in the health care professions: for example, its involvement in personal development, developing interpersonal skills and assisting with the feeling domains, widely used since the early deliberations of both Carl

Rogers and John Heron (Rogers, 1969; Heron 1977). Facilitation now forms an important part of the learning process and it is effective in providing a non-directive, non-confrontational flexible environment to assist student learning and development.

In practice the facilitator acts as a learning resource, creating the necessary climate for learning and offering guidance as required. Proficient facilitators are experienced and have patience to allow their students to be self-directive but are able to appreciate when their interventions are requested or needed (Wilkes, 1993). To promote effective learning, facilitative relationships have to be based on trust, respect and a genuine valuing of each other's abilities. It is clear that such a role fits well with the current ethos of adult learning.

General nursing, in particular, has experienced difficulties with the less positive elements of the clinical supervisor's role with the emphasis on admonishing and negative feedback. It would appear sensible to consider roles that combine the enabling aspects of facilitation with the practicalities of coaching functions. This could form the basis of a new direction for so called 'supervisory' learning support. Adding coaching functions could extend its meaning, for more general use and aid its acceptability as adult learning approaches and developing professional accountability continue to influence.

Coaching is perhaps a more acceptable concept for the 1990s with the health care challenges as new structures and different relationships develop. The modification to include coaching has been made primarily because the use of clinical supervision has fallen into disrepute because of its authoritarian overtones (Hill, 1989), but also, more positively, to acknowledge the new directions that learning as a developing professional is taking, in terms of the works of Schön (1988) and Barnet (1992). The concern that clinical supervision is no longer readily accepted tells us more about the nature of nursing than it does about the nature of supervision as a mechanism for developing and supporting students.

Nursing – confusion in roles

In British nursing and midwifery, mentoring has been used extensively but often inappropriately for student support and assessment – as will be discussed later in Chapter 3. Difficulties have arisen which will become readily apparent as you read through this book and the complexities of mentoring and preceptorship are unravelled.

Student nurses and student midwives now have access to personal tutors, are assessed by assessors, facilitated by mentors, and, in some instances all these complex roles with their individual responsibilities and possible conflicts are expected to be carried out by one qualified practitioner. In many cases the preparation is adequate but in others it is, at best, rudimentary, without exploration of the underpinning theoretical deliberations that are beginning to surface and be debated.

It can come as no surprise that there is lack of understanding and confusion with attempts made to bypass the real issues by inventing other labels. We have noted recently a rise in the different terms used for identifying those who support students through their educational programmes and practice placements. Besides the more readily recognizable labels already documented in this chapter, 'key worker', 'facilitator-aide', 'supporter', 'supervisor–mentor' are among the more interesting and colourful titles to be found. We could add one more to the growing list: that of the 'prementorceptor' an honorary title for those who are attempting to come to terms with being appointed as mentors! They are called mentors, function as preceptors, having to teach, support, assess and supervise students as they themselves, often in new posts, have to cope with the demands of their practice, having responsibilities for their own continuing professional development and by the nature of their caring profession, meeting the needs of patients, clients, customers or consumers. No wonder there is confusion.

It is time to address this confusing state of affairs by examining the range of support options available and setting the scene in order for sensible decisions to be made; sensible decisions made through effective communications between managers, practitioners, those concerned with initial student education, staff development and continuing professional education. If clinical supervision is unacceptable it may be more useful to draw on roles that provide support and offer guidance in the form of coaching, instruction and the use of positive feedback.

Sensitive handling and constructive debate is required on this support role as an appropriate mechanism for preparing professional practitioners in the early stages of their initial education and training programmes. It is our view that we should begin to look closely at the support that we provide for our students and to do that it is necessary to involve clinical practitioners, managers, researchers and educators. We should also start to define appropriate support systems that are applicable to the needs of those they are intended to benefit.

Coaching in health care

The term 'facilitator–coach' is chosen in the proposed support framework to encourage new ways of establishing student support within the required parameters of monitoring and assessment. The facilitator–coach concept draws on the two complementary roles of facilitation and coaching to enhance student learning and development in practice settings.

This term may appear as possibly contentious at this time of misused labels and roles. It has, however, been chosen in an attempt to widen the functions and responsibilities of the supervisor role, and to highlight the interactive, interpersonal processes that involve the acquisition of appropriate skills, actions and abilities that form the basis of professional practice. We see the role of facilitator–coach as instrumental in providing support for the student who is a new arrival to the profession and, as such, has specific needs and requirements.

'Coaching' is a relatively new term and it is one that may not rest easily in British health culture and nursing service domains. We believe it could be developed and used to reverse the negative connotations that surround the more readily recognizable support provided by supervision.

Coaching is a necessary prerequisite for students to develop effective skills and abilities within a supportive exchange of instruction, advice and positive feedback. Extending this role beyond its use in sport and business makes it necessary to adapt and clarify the functional elements of coaching – such as monitoring, assessment, instruction and feedback – in a manner that is conducive to the student entering a professional field of study and practice.

Here, the emphasis is on giving service and on caring. This wider interpretation of coaching places value on the humanistic theories of learning and contextual influences. Coaching, as described, can facilitate constructive monitoring and positive feedback of performance to assist the students to make sense of the professional world they are entering. Allowing students to set their own learning agendas, within flexible parameters of guidance and assistance, will encourage self-awareness and ensure that they take responsibility for their own learning needs which, in turn, are compatible with the standards expected.

The roles and responsibilities of the facilitator–coach

Coaching has been borrowed from the sporting world and is commonly found in commercial organisations where the emphasis is one of productivity and competition and where coaching relates to activities of team effort and achievement (Kelly, 1992).

Assisting with critical reflection

Reflection has become an educational 'buzz' word and Schön's (1988) view of the developing professional and critical reflection is helping to adjust the balances with theory and practice divisions. Indeed, it was Schön's work that raised the current interest in coaching and began the search to legitimize the use of the term in preparing new students for their professional working world. He used it to provide the guide to his 'virtual world', setting educators on the quest to identify the knowledge that underpins professional performance and informs on, in and through practice.

Based upon these interpretations, a facilitator–coach assists students to understand the nature of their role in professional practice and provides learning opportunities that allow the students to perform effectively.

The coach functions by setting the ground rules and offering instructions to the individual or team. These instructions are then carried out within a supervisory situation that is observed and can be reported upon. Discussion and feedback between those involved facilitates analysis and refinement of the practical efforts for future individual or team action.

This process involves working through problems, setting appropriate outcomes, carrying out mutually agreed actions, and is followed by recognition of what has been achieved by all those involved (Fournies, 1978). Offering positive, constructive feedback enhances the student's experiences because it is individual, unique to the student's requirements and it can allow the free exchange of ideas based on observations and mutually agreed outcomes.

The advice and counsel allows discussion of a particular situation or set of events. It implies close working relationships between facilitator–coach and the student. It also provides a setting for critical reflection and fits well with problem-solving approaches and experiential techniques. If used well and sensitively tuned to the student's needs, this facet of 'partnership in care' could go some way towards bridging the theory practice divide. It should also form one of the parts of a constructive plan for assisting the student to reflect in and on practice.

A checklist of key functions of the facilitator–coach

- Motivates students to set their own agendas for learning.
- Provides safe opportunities for learning.
- Advises, counsels and guides.
- Builds on a student's strengths by offering constructive feedback.
- Assists with students' progress in the practice placements.
- Provides an effective role-model.
- Assists students to learn through their successes and failures.

- Recognizes students' abilities and assesses their performance.
- Assists students to critically reflect on their practice.

The facilitator–coach can set standards but it is the student him-/herself who does it, and by the 'doing' is gaining the experience that can be reflected upon for future practice. In this manner students add to their repertoire of knowledge and experience and begin their entry to the profession.

Selection criteria for support roles – disabling and enabling strategies

Having established the need for support roles in the health service, it is important to consider the behaviours, qualities and characteristics of those who will be deemed suitable to provide the supportive role models for others. The intention is not to be prescriptive but to present some idea of what is meant by positive strategies in order to assist managers, educators and practitioners in making a sound selection. This will aid the deliberations of choosing who is best fitted to support others, who requires help in attaining appropriate qualities, and, perhaps also identify those who should never be placed in a position to support others.

In the chapters that follow a common theme in the discussion is the use of the term 'enabling' – epitomizing the positive aspects of human relationships that foster growth and development in others. 'Enabling' refers to the ability to make things happen, and in recent years it has become associated with the other positive development concepts of facilitation and empowerment. The working world would be a vastly different one if organizations were staffed and managed solely by people with these enabling qualities. The richness, complexity and challenges of the working culture is, however, diversified by the fact that human beings are capable of displaying both enabling and disabling qualities.

Disabling traits

In examining this aspect of the nature of support roles it is necessary to reflect on the less positive aspects of human nature which can have a detrimental effect on others.

Having identified individuals in management systems who are disruptive, Heirs & Farrell (1986) categorize these individuals whose thought processes and actions typify aspects of disabling behaviour. The 'destructive minds' are categorized by features as follows:

The rigid mind:
- Concrete thinkers, dealing with only black and white concepts.
- Stereotyped with preconceived ideas that are difficult to change.
- Set values, which lack imagination or creativity.
- In authority, stifle others, suspicious and resistant to new ideas.
- Safe and secure in bureaucratic surroundings.

The rigid mind: stifles originality, ignores change and encourages complacency.

The ego mind:
- Self-interested and self-important.
- Uninterested in others and keen to get their own way.
- Unable to share.
- Destroys team cohesiveness and spirit.
- Works well as an outsider or entrepreneur.

The ego mind: destroys objectivity and makes 'thinking collaboration' impossible.

The machiavellian mind:
- Devious and calculating, manipulative.
- Obsessed by internal politics and politicking'
- Interested in power and power plays.

The machiavellian mind: turns all thinkers into bureaucratic connivers and all thinking into political thinking.

Heirs & Farrell suggest that we should learn to manage these individuals and to attempt to understand how they operate. However, if this is not possible then their advice is to avoid them, taking care that they do not 'infect' your thinking (Heirs & Farrell, 1986, p. 86).

Vera Darling (1985), in taking a slightly different perspective offers a 'galaxy of toxic mentors', developed from interviewing nurses. Four distinct types of disabler are observed and these she refers to as the avoiders, dumpers, blockers and the destroyer/critizers. This informal classification and the associated sub-groups are presented in overview in Table 2.2. The apparent behaviours have similarities to those presented by the 'destructive minds'. These are clearly not the qualities expected of an enabler or those we would wish to identify as effective in supporting others. They present as those clearly at the other end of a continuum of positive supporting strategies.

Rather than present a continuum of positive support with polarizations of enabling and disabling traits which gives the appearance of being relatively simple and of one dimension, another positive attribute,

Table 2.2   The galaxy of toxic mentors.

Type	Features
Dumpers	Not available or accessible Throw people into new roles Leave them to 'sink or swim' strategies
Blockers	Avoid meeting others needs by: refusing requests ('the Refuser') controlling through withholding information ('the Withholder') arresting development by over supervising ('the Hoverer')
Destroyer/Criticizers	Set out to destroy others; categorized by: subtle attacks to undermine confidence ('the Underminer') open approaches of verbal attack and argument deliberate destroying confidence ('the Belittler') constant put-downs and questioning of abilities ('the Nagger')

Source: Darling (1985).

facilitation, can be added to the equation with that of another negative trait, such as manipulation. The resulting perspectives demonstrate the rich diversities of enabling and disabling characteristics that can occur.

This is demonstrated in Fig. 2.3. As can be seen, the positive qualities of enabling are in opposition to those of the negative disabling. These in turn are counter-balanced against the positive nature of facilitation and the negativity of manipulation.

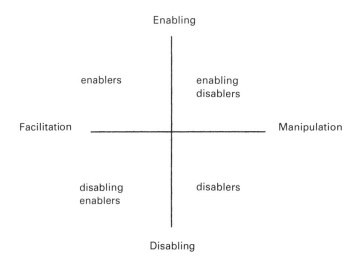

Fig. 2.3   Enabling–disabling traits.

This completes the four quadrants and the entities of the enablers, disablers and those that fall between, the enabling manipulator, (enabling-disabler) and disabling facilitator, (disabling-enabler) emerge. Although it is relatively easy to spot the true enablers and disablers within an organization, it is not always so easy to identify the negative and detrimental effects of those who are enabling-disablers or disabling-enablers. Often these individuals present with a much more subtle approach and it may take some time to realize that a relationship that appears as initially sound is disabling and having a negative effect.

The disablers fit with Darling's description of dumpers and blockers. The enabling-disablers and disabling-enablers are easily recognizable within the category of destroyers and criticizers. By creating tensions and disruptions, they can cause others to move departments or change jobs; conversely, enablers may create too comfortable an existence that is reassuring and seducing. That is not to say that these behaviours are tolerated, rather that an understanding of how they operate can help us work with, manage, and draw those who demonstrate disabling traits towards the beneficial effects of a supportive framework.

Enabling traits

Having dealt with the negative aspects we can now focus on the more positive elements. An enabler is someone who appears as an open, honest communicator, a person who feels positive about him/herself and about his/her value to the organization and to others within it.

Enablers are people-centred, and because they feel worthy and can value themselves, they are, in turn, able to recognize the value of others.

An enabling individual is:

- Accessible to those around him/her.
- Responsive to others' needs.
- Easy to trust.
- Comfortable with him-/herself and abilities.
- Able to command mutual respect.

Further discussions on enabling will be covered in detail in Chapters 3 and 4 as this is an important underlying feature of both mentoring and preceptorship. By recognizing the differing qualities, needs and aspirations of those around us, we can begin to assist them to remedy their limitations and value their strengths in becoming part of the team and providing support to others.

References

Ball, C. (1992) The Learning Society. *Royal Society of Arts Journal*, May, pp. 380–94.

Bandura, A. (1977) *Social Learning Theory*. Prentice-Hall, Englewood Cliffs, New Jersey.

Bandura, A. (1987) Analysis of modelling processes. In: *Contemporary Issues in Educational Psychology*. (Eds H.F. Clarizio, R.C. Craig & W.A Mehrens), pp. 158–62. Random House, New York.

Barber, P. & Norman, I. (1987) Skills in Supervision. *Nursing Times*, **83** (1) 56–7.

Barnett, R. (1990) *The Idea of Higher Education*. The Society for Research into Higher Education and the Open University.

Barnett, R. (1992) *Learning to Affect*. The Society for Research into Higher Education & OU Press, Buckingham.

Broome, A.K. (1990) *Managing Change*. Macmillan, Basingstoke.

Burnard, P. (1988) Self evaluation methods in Nurse Education. *Nurse Education Today*, **8**, 229–33.

Butterworth, T. (1992) Clinical Supervision as an Emerging Idea. In: *Clinical Supervision and Mentorship in Nursing*. (Eds T. Butterworth & J. Faugier), pp. 3–17. Chapman and Hall, London.

Butterworth, T. & Faugier, J. (Eds) (1992) *Clinical Supervision and Mentorship in Nursing*. Chapman and Hall, London.

Cormack, D.F.S. (ed) (1990) *Developing Your Career in Nursing*. Chapman Hall, London.

Daley, N.R. (1979) Burn out: smouldering problems in protective services. *Social Work*, **24**, 375–9.

Darling, V. (1985) What to do about toxic mentors. *The Journal of Nursing Administration*, May.

DoH (1989) *Working for patients*. Department of Health, HMSO, London.

DoH (1992) *The Citizen's Charter*. Department of Health, HMSO, London.

Earwaker, J. (1992) *Helping and Supporting Students. Rethinking the Issues*. The Society for Research into Higher Education, and The Open University.

Edwards, R. (1991) The inevitable future? Post-Fordism and open learning. *Open Learning*, June, 36–42.

Egan, G. (1990) *The Skilled Helper: A Systematic Approach to Effective Helping*. Brooks Cole Company, California.

Fournies, F.F. (1978) *Coaching for Improved Work Performance*. Van Nostrand Reinhold, New York.

George, J. (1986) Needed – care for carers. *The Health and Social Services Journal*, **96**, (13) 4980.

Gorz, A. (1989) *Critique of Economic Reason*. Verso, London.

Harvey, D. (1990) *The Condition of Postmodernity*. Blackwell Scientific Publications, Oxford.

Heirs, B. & Farrell, P. (1986) *The Professional Decision Thinker – Our New Management Priority* (2nd edition). Garden City Press Ltd, Hertfordshire.

Heron, J. (1977) *Dimensions of Facilitation Style.* Human Potential Research Project. Department of Adult Education. University of Surrey, Guildford.

Hill, J. (1989) supervision in the caring professions: a literature review. *Community Psychiatric Nursing Journal* **9**, (5) 9–15.

Hoggett, P. (1987) A farewell to mass production, in Hoggett, P. & Hambleton, R. (eds) *Decentralisation and Democracy.* SAUS, Bristol.

Johns, C. (1993) Professional supervision. *Journal of Nursing Management,* **1**, 9–18.

Kelly, K.J. (1992) *Nursing Staff Development, Current Competence Future Focus.* J.B. Lippincott, Philadelphia.

Kenworthy, N. & Nicklin, P. (1989) *Teaching and Assessing in Nursing Practice.* Scutari Press, Harrow.

Kolb, D.A. (1984) *Experiential Learning: Experience as the Source of Learning and Development.* Prentice-Hall, Englewood Cliffs, New Jersey.

London University (1992) *Roles and responsibilities of academic advisers,* in *Student Handbook, MA in Higher and Professional Education,* Centre for Higher Education Studies, London.

Marquis, B.L. & Huston, C.J. (1992) *Leadership Roles and Management Functions in Nursing: Theory and Application.* J.B. Lippincott, Philadelphia.

Murray, R. (1989) Fordism and Post-Fordism in Hull, S., Jacques, M. (eds). New Times: the Changing Face of Politics in the 1990s. Lawrence & Wisehart, London.

Oatley, K. & Johnson Laird, P.N. (1987) Towards a cognitive theory of emotions. *Cognition and Emotions,* **1**, 29–50.

Ogier, M. & Cameron-Buccheri, R. (1990) Supervision: a cross-cultural approach. *Nursing Standard,* **4** (31) 24–27.

Rogers, C.R. (1969) *Freedom to Learn.* Charles E. Merrill Publishing Co, Columbus, Ohio.

Ramsden, P. (1992) *Learning to Teach in Higher Education.* Routledge, London.

Rawlins, M.E. (1983) Mentoring and networking for helping professionals. *Personnel and Guidance Journal,* **62** (2) 116–118.

Rickards, T. (1992) *How to Win as a Mature Student.* Kogan Page, London.

Schön, D.A. (1988) *Educating the Reflective Practitioner: Towards a New Design for Teaching and Learning in the Professions.* Jossey-Bass, London.

Taylor, R.B. (1980) The role of the academic adviser. *Journal of Medical Education,* **55**: 216–217.

UKCC (1986) *Project 2000: A new Preparation for Practice,* United Kingdom Central Council, London.

UKCC (1993) *The Council's Position Concerning a Period of Support and Preceptorship for Nurses, Midwives and Health Visitors Entering or Re-Entering Registered Practice,* Annex One to Registrar's Letter 1/1993, United Kingdom Central Council, London.

Weil, S.W. & McGill, I. (Eds) (1989) *Making Sense of Experiential Learning: Diversity in Theory and Practice,* Society for Research into Higher Education and the Open University, Milton Keynes.

Wilkes, J. (1993) *Teacher/Facilitator: What's in a Title?* Nursing Times Open Learning notes, first draft, unpublished paper.

Wilkin, M. (1993) Initial training as a case of postmodern development: some implications for mentoring in McIntyre, D., Hagger, H. & Wilkin, M. (eds) *Mentoring: Perspectives on School-Based Teacher Education,* pp. 37–53. Kogan Page, London.

Chapter 3
Mentoring

'"Come to the edge", he said.
They said, "We are afraid".
"Come to the edge", he said.
They came.
He pushed them . . .
and they flew!'

Guillaume Apollinaire

What is mentoring?

This complex, intriguing concept has been taxing authors and researchers from a variety of different fields for many years. From its origins in classical Greece through business interpretations of the 1970s with adaptations in education and nursing during the 1980s, much has been written about the subject and a multitude of different approaches taken (Merriam, 1983).

Mentoring has become a high profile topic in business, women's magazines, the press and nursing, and it is beginning to re-emerge in current teacher-preparation initiatives. Mentoring has associations with the personal and professional development of individuals in a wide variety of organizational settings. It is also seen as a necessary factor for career socialization, advancement and success. Claims have been made that mentors:

- Make good leaders (Zaleznik, 1977)
- Are required for success in business (Collins & Scott 1978)
- Are needed for executive success (Roche, 1979)
- Lead to scholarliness (May *et al.*, 1982)
- Are a key to the future of nursing professionalism (Cooper, 1990)

Mentoring is indeed in vogue. Everyone has one or is beginning to want one. But is the concept clearly understood? What is a mentor? How do mentors function? What is mentoring? What are the complexities of the processes involved? These are questions that need to be addressed if appropriate and viable mentoring systems are to be developed. To separate out the myths from the mystique of mentoring is crucial, and one has to consider the origins, influences, approaches, terminology and the variety of different contexts in which mentoring has become viable in recent years.

Origins

The term 'mentor' is derived from the Classics, as identified in Homer's *Odyssey*. Mentor, the trusted son of Alimus, was appointed by Ulysses to be tutor–adviser to his son, Telemachus, and guardian of his estates while he was away fighting the Trojan wars. Mentor became more than a guardian, teacher and adviser. He had considerable influence and personal responsibility for the development of young Telemachus. Homer further informs that the goddess Athena assumed the disguise of Mentor to act as adviser to the youth. Safire (1980) suggests it was all a trick and that Homer was sending a warning to look out for mentors! It could be, however, that the poet was drawing attention to the complex nature of the relationship; the suggestion being that there was more to the role than that of an older, wiser, adviser of first impressions.

It was common in ancient Greece for young males to be partnered with older, experienced males. These were often relatives or friends of the family and it was expected that the youths would learn from and emulate the values of their assigned 'mentor'. The term 'mentor' thus became synonymous with wise, faithful guardian and teacher (Hamilton, 1981).

Roman generals had mentors by their side on the field of battle to advise them, and there are links with mentorship in the master craftsman–apprenticeship unions of mediaeval times. Guild masters were not only responsible for the teaching of particular crafts but also for their apprentices' social, religious and personal habits.

Few references to mentoring appear in the literature until a resurgence of interest in the concept was generated by Levinson's important study of adult development (Levinson *et al.*, 1978). The mentor was identified as ordinarily older, of greater experience and more senior in the world that the young man was entering. This mentor was viewed as a transitional, exemplar figure in a young male's development. This was built upon in business, education and nursing with the result that mentors and mentoring have been firing the imagination of many diverse occupational groups and professions in recent years (Vance, 1982).

Mentoring terms

The literature is full of various labels for the mentor and mentoree (the individuals involved) and mentoring or mentorship (the process). The identified labels within a structured, mentoring programme appear to reflect the organizational culture, management style, philosophy or mission of a particular organization. In health care it is more usual to find mentorees variously described as mentee or student. Murray & Owen (1991) document popular labels in other organizational settings as 'apprentice', 'aspirant', 'advisee', 'counselee', 'trainee protégé' and 'candidate'. Less popular terms used are 'follower', 'subordinate', 'applicant', 'hopeful', 'seeker' and we would add 'pupil', 'ward', 'novitiate' and 'initiate', which are limiting and judgemental when used in a mentoring context.

Influences

Moves towards providing organizational support systems that place importance on personal growth and development have roots in a variety of different movements of the 1970s and 1980s. The emergence of management theory and the role of management as a distinct discipline have played a part. However, the major influences appear to have been the human resource development initiatives of the 1970s (Eng, 1986), and the acceptance of freedom to learn approaches and adult learning theories, particularly Knowles (1984). The resulting shift in organizational and educational philosophies has led to the search for effective strategies that are directed towards making the most of human potential. The emphasis upon being self- directed and on *owning* the learning experience has increased responsibility for self-learning, self-awareness and problem-solving, which arises from the acceptance of the theoretical assumptions of adult development and maturation. This involves acknowledging that adults can:

- Move from a state of dependence to become self-directed – able to take responsibility for their own actions, self-development and life-long learning.
- Accumulate experiences – being able to build a biography of experience that can be drawn upon to test and evaluate new experiences. This, in turn, leads to the search for new learning opportunities, resulting in abilities to learn, change, and provide a rich resource for themselves and others.
- Have an orientation towards personal developmental and professional roles, demonstrating a willingness to learn and seek guidance as necessary.
- Change from needing to acquire content and being subject-centred to

becoming more performance-centred, resulting in the application of experience and the development of sound problem-solving abilities.

Underpinning these assumptions is the notion that individual growth is perceived as a process of becoming, and not as a process of being shaped or cloned. It is important to realize that self-experience and self-discovery are important facets of learning (Rogers, 1983). Adults have built-in motivations to learn, and a need to gain in self-confidence, self-esteem and self-awareness. These are important attributes for any occupational or professional group but crucial for those caring for the health needs of others. Self-awareness is also an important and necessary prerequisite for 'appreciating self and the situation of others' (Burnard, 1988, p. 229). This is a vital component of personal growth and development, it fits well with the 'process of becoming' as a continual journey of self-discovery. Assistance, offered by a confident, self-secure, experienced guide and enabler, in the form of a mentor, can aid the keen, inexperienced traveller.

The *raison d'être* of mentoring

Mentoring is an exciting complex phenomenon that is natural or artificially contrived to benefit individuals within a sharing partnership (Palmer, 1987). In the true Classical sense it is much more than the experienced guiding the inexperienced: mentoring is dynamic and exciting – in part because of its kaleidoscopic nature and also because it is a relatively complex concept, made intricate by the various connotations placed upon it. It is a good example of a transcendental semantic signifier – taken in this context to mean that mentoring can be viewed from many different perspectives and is open to a variety of interpretations, depending on its differing applications and settings.

Mentoring concerns the building of a dynamic relationship in which the personal characteristics, philosophies and priorities of the individual members interact to influence, in turn, the nature, direction and duration of the resulting, eventual partnership. What lies at the heart of the process is the shared, encouraging and supportive elements that are based on mutual attraction and common values. It is these aspects that facilitate the personal development and career/professional socialization for the mentoree – leading to eventual reciprocal benefits for both parties.

A mentoring relationship is one that is enabling and cultivating; a relationship that assists in empowering an individual within the working environment. A mentor is not a prerequisite for advancement or success – such events regularly occur without access to this type of significant helper. Mentors do not have magic abilities or powers to fashion great individuals (Fields, 1991). They do, however, enable individuals to discover and use their own talents, encouraging and nurturing the unique contributions of their mentorees, to assist them to be successful in their own right.

Mentoring is concerned with making the most of human potential, and it is significant that it has become more widely recognized in health care at a time of restricted resources and moves towards managed markets. As part of an identified support framework of other, more recognizable roles, and staff development programmes, mentoring fits well with humanistic management, education, and training initiatives. This involves adult approaches and learning experiences, supported by the principles of self-development, self-directedness, mutual understanding, and negotiation.

However, in the British health service and education system, currently concerned with market economies, efficiency and value-for-money, mentoring mechanisms of a more formalized nature may rest more easily with the prevailing ethos. For the clinical manager, educator, staff developer or researcher mentoring presents as an intriguing challenge when considering the what, how and where of practical application.

Mentoring challenges

On examining mentoring, it becomes apparent that the views from a variety of perspectives and the lack of clarity of purposes and functions of the mentor are not assisted by anecdotal reports, lack of empirical evidence and confusion with other support roles. What is crucial in today's climate is a need to come to terms with the nature of new support roles and to then apply them appropriately. This is important with regard to the types of approaches that are available and may be required.

Important questions to be considered include who needs, wants or will benefit from such new roles? Making informed decisions about what systems are required, how they should be planned, implemented, evaluated and resourced will enable managers, educators and those from staff development units to make adequate preparations to assist staff to come to terms with the new support roles, structures and frameworks.

It would be easy to step into the quagmire of definitions, envisaged by Hagerty (1986). It is far better to clarify the roles that already exist and to consider the nature of the classical mentor as interpreted by Levinson *et al.* (1978). This leads to the discovery of the richness of the relationship and facilitates an explanation of the various mentoring approaches that are available. The informed decisions and choices can then be made regarding the development of sound mentoring mechanisms to complement the other organizational support systems that are available.

The classical mentor

Common elements underpin the different perspectives, cultures and approaches. Vance (1982) helps to clarify the situation by drawing attention to the earlier suggestions arising from business studies, that mentoring is not defined in the identification of formal roles but in the character of the relationship and the function it serves. Business, education and nursing applications of mentoring may initially appear different in terminology, focus and approach. However, certain common elements emerge. These can be identified as:

- The character of the relationship is that of enabling and empowerment;
- The mentor offers a repertoire of helper functions (or assisting functions) to facilitate guidance and provide support;
- The mentor role comprises personal, functional and relational aspects;
- Individual purposes and helper functions are mutually set by the individuals involved;
- Helper functions are mutually determined by the individuals;
- Individuals choose each other and there are identifiable stages in the relationship.

Character of the relationship

In classical mentoring the central focus of the partnership concerns the mutual trust of two adult individuals attracted by the possibility of what has been described as a mentor signal (George & Kummerow, 1981). The two parties are drawn together naturally by their personal characteristics, attributes and common values. They demonstrate a willingness to spend time together, to learn from each other and to share each other's experiences.

In the early stages of the relationship the mentoree may appear dependent or reliant on the mentor in terms of the intensity of the support offered. As the relationship develops this intensity will change as the needs and priorities of the mentoree change. This results in an intimacy to the relationship made possible by mutual relevance and closeness. A partnership develops into one that is dynamic, reciprocal, and emotionally intense.

Recognition of the partnership, and better understanding his/her own needs allows the mentoree to become proactive in triggering the specific support or assistance required. The mentoree can begin to be self-selecting with regard to the helper functions required and begin to make informed decisions about personal development.

Testing, taking risks, making mistakes, and the freedom to be creative takes place within the mutual understanding that the mentoree is valued and supported. Safety mechanisms exist in the form of the wide range of helper functions offered by the mentor. The mentoree becomes gradually more self-aware, gains in confidence and begins to achieve the capacity to 'go it alone'. It is at this stage that she or he may look for another mentor or become a mentor to someone else.

In this manner the classical mentor facilitates personal growth and development, and assists with career development while guiding the mentoree through the clinical, educational, social and political networks of the working culture. The aspects of mentoring that set it apart from other, more specific relationships to give it its multidimensional and dynamic nature are the:

- Repertoire of helper functions.
- Mutuality and reciprocal sharing.
- Duration, identified stages and transitional nature of the relationship.

These required elements match those of Darling (1984) who maintains that the vital ingredients for mentoring are attraction, action and effect.

Repertoire of helper functions

Within work, individuals may develop relationships that are specific in nature such as role modelling or teaching. These relationships are clearly defined and are functionally specific. If a deeper association develops with mutual attraction, and the wide range of helper functions are offered, then the relationship becomes one that is dynamic, reciprocal, emotionally intense and true, classical mentoring occurs (Palmer, 1987, p. 36). The emotional aspect arises from an intimacy that is made possible by the closeness and understanding of those involved. The helper functions of mentoring are:

- Adviser
- Coach
- Counsellor
- Guide/networker
- Role model

- Sponsor
- Teacher
- Resource facilitator

Adviser

Support and advice is offered in both career and social terms. The advice given demonstrates an awareness of the mentoree's merits and abilities within the organization's requirements. This process aids in building image and confidence of the mentoree.

Coach

In mentoring the coaching function concerns the mutual setting of guidelines with the mentor offering advice and instruction. The mentoree can test such instruction in differing practice situations. The mutual exchange between the individuals allows feedback to be analysed and refined for future action.

Counsellor

This facilitates self-development of the mentoree in his/her own terms; psychological support systems are made available. The mentor acts as a listener and sounding-board to facilitate self- awareness and encourage independence.

Guide/networker

As a supportive guide, the mentor introduces the mentoree to the helpful contacts and power groups within the organization. Networking is an extension of guiding: the mentor facilitates introductions to the values and customs of the organization to include socialization to the mentor's own occupational, professional and social groups.

Role model

This provides an observable image for imitation, demonstrating skills and qualities for the mentoree to emulate.

Sponsor

This influences and facilitates entry to the organizational and professional culture. Influences career by providing introductions, promoting the mentoree and making recommendations for advancement.

Teacher

This involves sharing knowledge through experience and inquiry, facilitating learning opportunities and focusing on individual needs and learning styles to promote ownership and responsibility for continuing education. It assists in personal development in order to fulfil intellectual and practical potential.

Resource facilitator

The mentor acts as an experienced practitioner and colleague sharing experiences and information, and providing access to resources. This forms the preceptor-type element of the helper functions.

Personal, functional and relational factors

The personal and relational factors are concerned with individual growth, development, self-awareness and fulfilment. Knowing that there is someone there willing to offer support and encouragement and 'in their corner', enables the mentoree to come to terms with his/her role in the organization or professional setting. The mentor offers personal, functional and relational assistance to provide a framework of support. Within such a framework the mentoree can begin to constructively question his/her own abilities, gain in confidence, be creative and endeavour to take risks. The inter-relationship of these personal, functional and relational factors are identified in Table 3.1.

Table 3.1 The support framework of personal, functional and relational factors within mentoring.

| | Mentor role | |
Personal	Functional	Relational
promoting:	*providing:*	*facilitating:*
Self-development	Teaching	Interpersonal relations
Confidence building	Coaching	Social relations
Creativity	Role modelling	Networking
Fulfilment of potential	Counselling	Sharing
Risk-taking	Support	Trust
	Advice	
	Sponsorship	
	Guidance	
	Resources	

Mutual setting of individual purposes and functions

Jointly attracted by each other's qualities and attributes, in classical mentoring the mentor and mentoree are free to develop the relationship in the manner of their choosing. The emphasis is on informality. The needs of the individuals concerned form the character and nature of the resulting relationship. The mentoree can feel safe in selecting helper functions that are required in his/her own terms, while moving from initial dependency in the relationship to becoming independent and his/her own person.

In classical mentoring informal assessment may exist in the tentative, early phases of the partnership but only in the form of evaluating each other's experiences, abilities, approachability and willingness to give time. Formal assessment and documentation procedures have no place in classical mentoring.

Mentor language, functions and organizational culture

In classical mentoring the nature and terms of the relationship are set informally by the people involved. The nature of the relationship is determined by the qualities and characteristics of the people drawn together by common values or attitudes to form an initial attraction. The processes which evolve are mutually formulated by both parties, naturally occurring and informal within the specific organizational culture. The expectations and any issues that arise will relate to what the mentor and mentoree may deem as important in gaining the 'tribal wisdom' of an organization (Darling, 1984) or obtaining the 'DNA of a profession' (Palmer, 1992).

The expectations include the need for active participation and developmental outcomes tailored to the needs of the mentoree to provide a sharing, collaborative partnership that benefits both individuals, the organization or relevant occupational group, or profession.

The nature of the relationship will be affected by the organizational culture which consists of the values, norms, and beliefs of the structures and systems that give an organization its own identity (Handy, 1985). In classical mentoring the relationship is inherently of their own making. Modifications to classical mentoring in order for it to fulfil a variety of differing individual and organizational requirements has led to the application of more formal approaches. The true elements of classical mentoring, (mutuality, repertoire of helper functions, duration) may well be evident but there will be adaptations and a differing emphasis placed on career support, socialization and criteria for success.

Mentoring and Preceptorship

In more formal forms of mentoring such as contract, (Monaghan & Lunt, 1992) or facilitated mentoring (Murray & Owen, 1991), mentor terminology and helper functions are determined by the organizational culture (see Table 3.2 for an explanation of approaches). Contract mentoring concerns the adaptation of classical mentoring and its resulting application within structured programmes. The people involved are obliged to achieve the identified aims, purposes and outcomes of a recognized programme of development and support. The relevant aims, purposes and outcomes may, or may not, be negotiable,

Table 3.2 Mentoring approaches.

Mentoring type	Features
1. True mentoring relationships	
(i) Classical mentoring/Informal (primary mentoring) A natural, chosen relationship. Purposes and functions are determined by the individuals involved. An enabling relationship in personal, emotional, organisational and professional terms.	• self-selection of individuals, persuasive influences; attraction with a shared wish to work together; • No defined programme; • Less specific purposes and functions as set by the individuals, circumstances and context; • No explicit financial rewards for mentor; • Lengthy duration, 2–15 years.
(ii) Contract mentoring/Formal (Facilitated mentoring/Secondary mentoring) An artificial relationship created for a specific purpose, that is essentially determined by the organisation. Some elements of mentor function, with focus on specific helper functions.	programmes are identified by: • Clear purposes, functions, defined aims or outcomes; • Selected individuals with assigned mentors, forced matching or choice of mentors from mentor pool; • Explicit material rewards; possibilities of financial incentives for mentors; • Shorter duration, 1–2 years.
2. Pseudomentoring relationships (Quasi mentoring/partial mentoring/ sequential mentoring) Mentoring approaches in appearance only – as offered by academic involvement in thesis preparation, orientation and induction programmes.	• Focus on specific tasks or organizational issues of short lived duration; • Guidance from several mentors, for short periods; • Relationships do not demonstrate the comprehensive enabling elements of the true classical model; • Specified clinical placements; • Short duration 6 weeks to one year.

depending on the degree of formality of the programme. Individuals can be assigned to each other (forced matching) or may be able to make a choice from a selected group of mentors, known as the 'mentor pool'.

The nature of the process may have superficial similarities within different organizations or within differing occupational groups but how the process is explained and understood may take on a variety of appearances. Often formulated for organizational requirements as part of staff development programmes, the use of different terminology and the change in emphasis for the helper functions give rise to the different approaches of mentoring that are evident within differing cultures.

Classical mentoring and contract mentoring can be considered as true mentoring as both contain the vital elements essential to mentoring; these being the helper functions, mutuality and sharing, and identified stages/duration. Pseudo- mentoring of quasi-mentoring approaches have probably occurred due to the initial lack of understanding of the roles, purposes, processes and formal applications of mentoring.

Early applications tended to confuse mentoring with the support provided by preceptors, academic counsellors and personal tutors. Mentoring was also used for the singular purposes of orientation and induction. (An elaboration of quasi-mentoring is offered in Table 3.2.)

Organizational applications in business and education

In business, the emphasis is for the mentor to function as a sponsor, guide or networker within a competitive culture that is often male-dominated. The main focus has been on career guidance, executive nurturing and managerial support, with informal or formal, planned programmes of contract/facilitated mentoring (Murray & Owen, 1991).

In the USA, business interest in mentoring systems stimulated education policy-makers and educators to consider such approaches for student preparation, teachers and school administrators (Fagan & Walter, 1982; Klopf & Harrison 1981). The focus for mentor function was that of teacher and role model, the educational aims being adapted from those of business to reduce the accent on financial rewards. Education has become more concerned with product and process, resulting in roles for educators that simulate adult learning and alter the power of learning towards the student.

In education in the UK, the focus for mentoring programmes was initially conceived for educational and pastoral support in probationary periods. Scant further interest being taken in the concept, despite the recommendations of the James Committee (1972). Later, in the 1970s, the Advisory Committee on the Supply and Training of Teachers

(ACSTT) set up a sub-committee, chaired by Professor Haycocks which subsequently produced three influential reports. The second sub-committee report on the training of adult education and part-time further education teachers (ACSTT II), which became more popularly known as Haycocks II, reported in March 1978.

One of the reports' recommendations centred on the provision of a local team of mentors to offer roles as classroom counsellors in teacher training. Holt (1982, p. 153) in valuing such a proposal for 'on course, in house support', identified difficulties in implementation because of cost, mentor training and the effectiveness of the supervisory role in the classroom. Beyond initial school education, the envisaged changes had implications for general staff development, providing 'training for the trainers' and for those involved in further education, (Cantor & Roberts, 1986, p. 192). Current interest has once again arisen due to the envisaged changes in initial teacher training programmes, (Department for Education, 1992). Student teachers are to be based in educational placements and to learn 'on the job', with support from a qualified teacher acting as a mentor.

Application to health care

In British health care, supportive role developments have been many and varied. Occupational groups, such as social workers and occupational therapists, have structured, sound, clinical enabling relationships that develop therapeutic competence (Hawkins & Shohet, 1989), that assist training, and also facilitate assessment in practical placements. Modifications of therapeutically determined supervisory roles, allow learning support to be provided by practising field-work teachers, supervisors and community trainers. Those in physiotherapy also recognize a need for students to experience professional work, enabling them to re-examine practice effectively through investigation, analysis and support (Pratt, 1989).

Further information of how these and other health occupations provide learning support will be forthcoming from research currently in progress. A two-year study being carried out by The Open University (building upon work previously undertaken by the now-disbanded Council for National Academic Awards) has been funded by the Department of Employment. The project team, led by Dr Nigel Nixon, is considering the development of students' subject area knowledge and skills in work-based components of higher education programmes. The subject areas being investigated are health and social sciences, computing and mathematics, engineering and technology, as well as art, design and the performing arts. The team have commenced the case-study phase which will examine different approaches to work-based learning and the learning-support role. The national report is due for publication in the autumn of 1994 (Nixon & Fenwick, 1993).

In British nursing and midwifery, mentoring issues have been further complicated with the confusion over the role and functions of other support roles, namely that of preceptors. A few mentor programmes for senior managers were instigated in the early 1980s and 'faculty mentors' were recommended in training medical students (Calkins, *et al.*, 1987; Muller, 1984). For the most part in the health service at present, mentoring is 'provided' for student nurses and student midwives.

It is well-documented that the terms 'mentor' and 'preceptor' were bought to the consciousness of most British nurses via the educational language and curriculum development of the last decade. The nursing originators who set the scene for the take up of the concept in the UK were mainly North American authors, consultants and researchers notably Vance (1982) Darling (1984) and Puetz (1985). Most admit to having drawn on the experiences of the business and commercial arenas where the empirical evidence has involved mostly male experiences in the world of work.

Nursing, midwifery and the other professions allied to medicine remain primarily female-dominated and transferring empirical and anecdotal evidence from different cultures can further complicate understanding and application. There are fundamental differences of product-process ethos between business and service organizations like the health service which has imperatives for setting social objectives – 'managing for social result' (Weil, 1992). In nursing, important mentoring issues of cross-gender approaches and some female nurses' lack of apparent abilities to network, share and support emerging leaders has been readily addressed, (Hamilton, 1981; Hardy, 1984).

The word 'mentor' first appeared in the curriculum preparation documents produced by one of the statutory bodies, the English National Board (ENB, 1987; 1988). New roles were rapidly created and new name badges worn with some pride and a great deal of puzzlement for both qualified staff and students alike. The use of the term 'preceptor' – again with its origins in North America – had appeared earlier in the nursing index for 1975 and in popular nursing press reports, where a scheme was supposedly developed within one health authority (Raichura & Riley, 1985).

The use of preceptors has once again been bought to the attention by the stated intentions of PREPP (UKCC, 1990) and examination by British authors and researchers (Morle, 1990; Barlow, 1991). Nursing authors have switched from discussing the merits of mentorship to comparing and contrasting the merits of both roles and how they could best be used (Armitage & Burnard, 1991; Ashton & Richardson, 1992).

Clarity about the nature of the different roles has not been helped by early articles that attempted to describe mentoring that, with the benefit of hindsight, were describing preceptorship programmes of quasi-mentoring approaches. Morle (1990) concluded that current role definition is probably inappropriate and nursing would be better advised to use the term 'preceptor' – a role more orientated and suited to practice. What is important in the current debate is that mentoring and preceptorship should be seen to have equal value for development and support in whichever setting they are applied.

Choice and mentoring stages

Individual selection is a vital process of classical mentoring. The relationship is dependent on the joint, dynamic, sharing, characteristics of both parties for its nature and success. Matching characteristics and a 'coming together' are naturally implied in the mentor signal and common attraction that ignites the relationship. Enjoyment of each other's company and a willingness to spend time together may signal the start to this informal mentoring process. Styles of approach and the individual preferences of both parties play their part in how the 'personal fit' is made (Klopf & Harrison, 1981).

Phases or stages to the relationship are variously described and documented (Campbell-Heider, 1986). The phases are commonly identified as the initiation, development, and termination. Hunt & Michael (1983) suggest that there are four phases and identify these as: initiation, training, and termination, with the establishment of lasting peer friendship as a follow-up to an amicable ending.

Other writers specify invitational, questioning, informational/working and termination stages (Hawkins & Thibodeau, 1989). What is common to many of the deliberations on the phases or stages, is that there is always a recognizable start, middle and end to the relationship.

Initiation

The start or initiation, concerns the 'locking on' of individuals who are brought together by common characteristics, abilities, or recognition of similar value systems. This involves the selection and 'getting to know you' period of the relationship. Working in close proximity, having access to each other and being able to observe each others' actions in a variety of work situations, influences the initial attraction and assists the start.

Working phase

The working or training phase of the process is where the main focus for individual growth and development lies. The dynamics of the mentoring relationship are maintained by the joint interactions of both individuals and the increasing trust and closeness that begins to develop. The mentoree may start this phase by being heavily reliant upon the mentor's greater experience, and awareness of the networks and wide variety of influential contacts.

The mentoree is faced with the repertoire of helper functions that the experienced mentor has to offer and the choice of assistance may initially be erratic and left to chance. As this phase develops, mutual trust and sharing becomes evident and the mentoree is more readily able to choose the helper functions that are best suited to his/her needs. This is a very active phase, and the intensity of the relationship moves to that of common understanding and solid partnership. The mentoree gradually becomes more independent and is eventually able to trigger or request the specific helper functions required.

Through the mutual sharing of experiences and needs, the mentoree is able to make informed decisions and become self-selecting within the

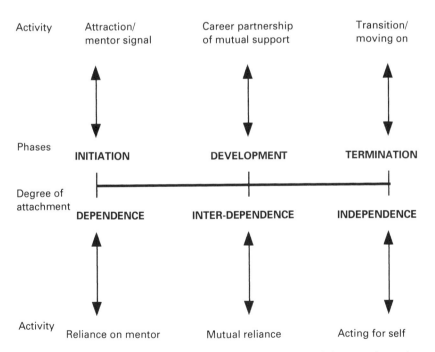

Fig. 3.1 Matching phases of mentoring with activities and degree of attachment. (Adapted Palmer, 1987.)

relationship. Fig. 3.1 shows the mentoring phases with activities and degree of attachment. This sets the scene for the mentoree to have the confidence to be creative, and to experiment with risk-taking ventures that further encourage growth.

The need to test and take risks arises within the understanding that the mentoree is valued, supported and that there are safety measures available should mistakes occur. The mentoree becomes increasingly more confident to 'go it alone' and the relationship moves towards the terminating phase.

Termination phase

The mentoree has begun to act on his/her own initiative and is now in a position to begin to act independently. The termination phase can end positively as supportive friendship or negatively where there is conflict or emotional tension and general dissatisfaction (Blotnick, 1984; Wheatley & Hirsch, 1984). The ending can be precipitated by changing career interests, a need to find another mentor, to take on the challenges of mentoring others or the results of toxic mentoring. (This is explored more fully in the benefits and limitations of mentoring which follow later in this chapter.)

If the process has been beneficial with the identified needs being met, the two individuals may maintain their friendship and the mentoree may move on to mentor others. This may be due in part to the need for another association that involves sharing or a desire for the degree of emotional intensity that is not always readily available within ordinary working contacts.

Attributes, qualities and abilities of an effective mentor

Just as there is no single definition for that of the mentor, there is no single personality type that is synonymous with that of being or becoming an effective mentor. What is evident is that successful mentors are reported as employing a range of enabling strategies and skills within mentoring relationships (Fields, 1991). Other authors and researchers list an extensive range of characteristics or qualities that appear to be best suited to this type of long-term, close working relationship.

Extensive lists and tables of the essential ingredients to function as an effective mentor can be drawn together within a framework of three important personal attributes. These are competence, demonstrating personal confidence, and having a commitment to the development of others. In possessing these personal attributes the mentor has the qualities and abilities to extend a working relationship beyond that of ordinary limits to ensure that mentoring occurs and is effective for all concerned.

Competence

The mentor has competence:

- Arising from having the appropriate knowledge and experience to be effective in his/her work within the organization, and able to command respect from others.
- To build on the mentoree's strengths and offer constructive feedback on his/her limitations.
- In the skills associated with the repertoire of helper functions, such as interpersonal relations, communication, counselling, instructing and coaching; skills that are more valuable if exercised and up to date.
- In providing a reliable source of information and availability of resources.
- To promote good judgement.

Confidence

The mentor has confidence to:

- Have and share a network of valuable personal contacts.
- Be imaginative.
- Demonstrate initiative, take risks and have personal power with charisma that is used appropriately.
- Allow the mentoree to develop within his/her own terms.
- Seek new challenges and initiatives.
- Be successful at what she/he does, providing status and prestige.
- Lead and offer clear direction.
- Share credit of achievements.
- Be able to deal with another's personal problems, challenges and triumphs.

Commitment

The mentor is committed to:

- Staff development.
- Being people-orientated and having a keen interest in seeing others develop and advance.

- Investing time, energy and effort with a different type of working relationship.
- Sharing personal experiences, knowledge and skills.
- Personal motivation and a desire to motivate others.

Competence, confidence and commitment ensure that the mentor can be flexible, proactive and responsive to balance the requisites of a long-term, intimate working relationship with an understanding of its transitional nature and eventual conclusions.

It is also important that the mentor is self-aware with a clear sense of his/her own strengths and limitations, enabling assistance in another's personal growth and development. Positive qualities of flexibility, approachability, accessibility, political astuteness, patience, perseverance, and a sense of humour are also essential for effective mentorship. These are sound qualities that ensure that mentors are relatively at ease with themselves, do not take themselves too seriously and can with competence, confidence and commitment be generous towards others, playing their part as enabler and leader.

Qualities for attracting a mentor

Mentoring concerns two interested parties. Although the qualities and skills that a mentor possesses are vital to the nature and effectiveness of the ensuing relationship, the qualities of a mentoree also come into play when considering the unfolding of the relationship. The essential ingredients and basic roles to be undertaken are also influenced by the qualities, skills and characteristics of the linking mentoree. Indeed there are those who suggest that there are identifiable strategies that can be employed in attracting a mentor (Zey, 1984; p. 175).

Qualities that endeavour to make a mentoree potentially 'attractive' to a mentor include the following:

Standing out of the crowd:
- achieving high visibility,
- having a positive attitude to work or career,
- willing to take risks.

Demonstrating the potential to succeed:
- willingness to learn and assist the mentor to achieve goals,
- having initiative and being motivated,
- ambitious and conscientious,
- receptive to coaching and instruction.

Adult intimacy capabilities:
- having a positive self-esteem,
- able to make a personal contribution,
- loyal to individuals and the organization,
- enlightened and enthusiastic,
- making oneself accessible.

Benefits and limitations of mentoring

The benefits

The positive effects are mutually split to benefit the mentor, mentoree and organization (Zey, 1984; Cooper, 1990).The strengths and benefits of mentoring arise from the attraction, sharing, and developing properties of the relationship. The beneficial effects can be related to degrees of satisfaction for those involved:

> *the mentor:* personal satisfaction from aiding and abetting another's development;
> *the mentoree:* job satisfaction and possibilities of advancement and success as they become socialized to the organization;
> *the organization:* a satisfied and motivated workforce with positive outcomes for customers and clients.

Other benefits concern leadership development: qualities and abilities associated with mentoring are synonymous with effective leadership. Mentoring can assist in developing leaders with mentorees looked upon as emerging leaders, cultivated for their flexibility, adaptability, sound judgement and creativity within an organization.

Finally, thoughts should be directed towards the possible constraining factors that may inhibit mentoring from occurring, even if formal programmes of contract mentoring are organized. If mentoring is appropriately recognized as part of the organizational culture, working relationships are very likely to be more open and effective. Such openness improves communication and encourages a greater degree of collegiality and general sharing approaches.

The limitations

The limitations to mentoring are perhaps best described by the use of the term 'toxic mentoring', identified by Darling (1986). This concerns the disabling elements and strategies that may be employed by an ineffective mentor and these should be avoided at all cost.

The essence of toxicity arises from a relationship that is not built on mutual trust. Here, the mentoree is directed not facilitated, and disabled not enabled. It can take the form of an exploitative, manipulative relationship, the 'drone worker–bee syndrome' illustrated by Hawkins & Thibodeau (1989). Features of toxic mentoring are:

- The mentor uses the mentoree and does not promote the mentoree's ideas, taking any credit due.
- Some recognition of a partnership but the mentor uses the mentoree's abilities to further his/her own career and standing in the organization.
- The power in the relationship may remain with the mentor, resulting in mentoree manipulation, overprotection, dependency, and lack of development.
- Control and excessive direction causing the mentoree to conform to an identical set image of the mentor, resulting in cloning.
- Elitism and mutual seclusion causing the mentoree to withdraw from other relationships and become dependent on the mentor.

Strategies for avoiding toxic mentors

(1) Self-select a classical mentor or if offered a mentor programme, choose a mentor who is interested and who can be worked with.
(2) Do not choose an individual who is a disabler.
(3) Examine the relationship regularly for signs of toxicity – cloning, dependency; mentor self interest, manipulation or exploitation.
(4) Monitor personal development and prepare a sound, appropriate end to the relationship
(5) Be prepared to eject from a mentor who is showing signs of toxicity.
(6) Ensure that the person chosen as a mentor is successful and 'going places' in the organization.

Recognition of the benefits and limitations of mentoring facilitates a better understanding of what mentoring is all about and allows a healthy dialogue to commence regarding the salient issues that may arise.

Constraints to mentoring

Although personnel newly appointed to an organization may have the necessary personal qualities for mentoring, they are initially unlikely to have the networking contacts to provide for effective mentoring. However, as they settle into the organization culture they will lack power, experience and influence within the organisation.

Other constraints to effective mentoring – particularly classical mentoring – are working cultures where there is a rigid hierarchy or where disabling strategies prevail. Clutterbuck (1985) further identifies problems in organizations where heavy politics are evident, staff turn-over is high and poor morale act as deterrents to effective mentoring.

Mentoring limitations of working cultures where women make up the majority of the work force, and how this affects whether mentoring exists or not are well documented by writers exploring the nature of mentoring (Hardy, 1984; May *et al.*, 1982, p. 27). It is important to note that in nursing, midwifery and other professional groups where most of the working population is female, there are issues of gender that ought to be taken into account.

Women's working image and self-esteem, along with the training and education of women professional groups, and their socialization into vocational work, have to be further explored and researched. Whilst there is evidence for constraints, such as women having to manage alone and having little time or effort left to support others, there is growing evidence that women do indeed identify with the need to support and bring others along as they make their own way through corporate and professional environments. Vance (1979) suggests that women do help and support each other, even if they do not formally recognize this assistance as mentoring. Although not always recognizing or fully appreciating the networking qualities of the processes involved, Sheehy (1976) reported that 'women who haven't had a mentor relationship miss it, even if they don't know what to call it' (Sheehy, 1976, p. 34). The confusion about mentoring over the years has added to the difficulties of recognition and this comment could apply equally well to men.

However, when considering women and mentoring, it is important to appreciate the issues of language, organizational context and sexual stereotyping in formulating, reflecting and reinforcing ideologies of gender (Parsons, 1993). Formal mentoring programmes constructed from business-orientated models may indeed offer a foundation for design but should be adapted to encompass readily the working needs of women in health care.

Formal mentoring: devising a mentor programme

In setting up a mentor programme, with the notion of providing formal mentoring, supplying contract mentors or facilitated mentors, it is important to appreciate the complexities involved. Whether the decision is made to build your own programme or to buy in 'ready-made, adapted-to-fit-your-needs programmes' the groundwork has to be thorough and the intentions clear if the venture is to be a success. For diagrammatic representation of a workable model for practice see Fig. 3.2, which presents an overview; Fig. 3.3 shows the processes involved.

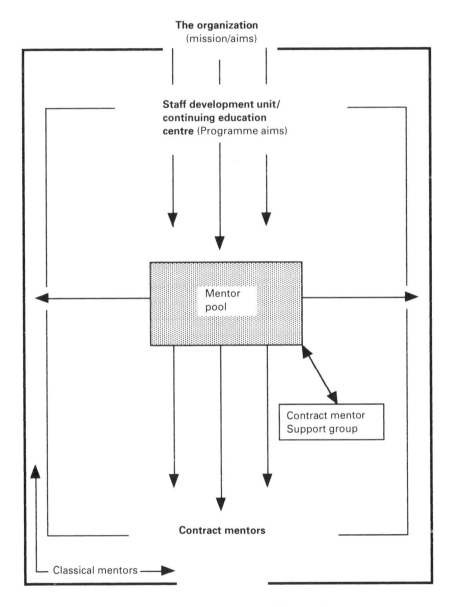

Fig. 3.2 Formal mentoring – A workable model for practice, an overview.

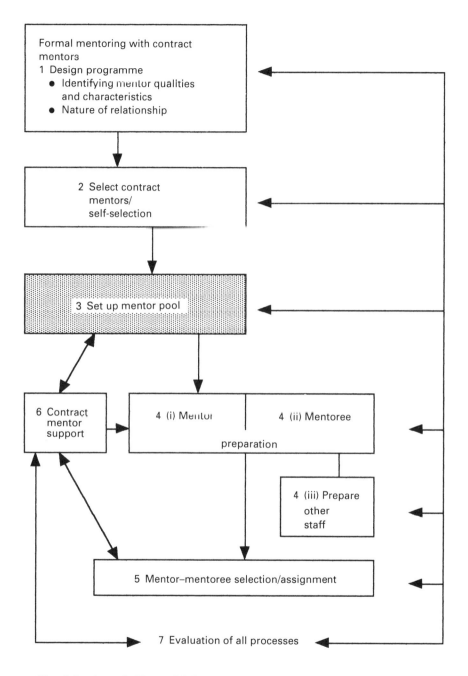

Fig. 3.3 A workable model for practice: processes involved in formal mentoring.

Design deliberations should include:

- The type of mentoring approaches to be employed.
- Resource allocation.
- Mentor–mentoree preparation and support.
- Effective evaluation.

Resources and approaches

This will depend on the requirements of the organization, what is available and the commitment of senior staff for this type of support development. A general shift towards an appreciation that a learning culture is good for staff, customers and business has led to motor manufacturers providing increased resources for staff development (Ball, 1992). Those interested in developing mentoring programmes within the health service can draw on the experiences of these other organizations to convince managers that effective investment in sound programmes will have an impact on staff with the ultimate aim of improving patient/client care. There is increasing evidence that mentoring is effective as part of a recognizable staff development programme and that it benefits working relationships (Kelly, 1992).

Sensible resource decisions also require consideration of the types of approaches to be used. It is uneconomical to devise intricate formal mentoring structures with extensive mentor preparation if all that is required is staff induction and orientation. Of course these elements can be incorporated into the contract mentoring role, but it will not be cost-effective if the process required is someone to introduce new staff or someone to acclimatize returners. This can be readily incorporated into existing management roles.

Similarly a preceptor model may be more appropriate if used in its original sense for students, where functions and roles are determined by short learning placements with supervision with assessment. Preceptorship may also be useful in clinical staff development, where staff are qualified and changing position or departments. However, it should be noted that in British nursing the nature of preceptorship has been adapted by the UKCC (1990), who has advised that it be used for specific staff preparation and transition periods.

Effective economies can be made by shared learning opportunities or by including mentor preparation in other programmes focusing on interpersonal, facilitation and enabling skills. Preceptors and mentors can be prepared together for part of a common programme, as long as the similar elements and differences are made very clear. This should work well in aiding understanding of each other's role. It will also help to start the 'mutual respect and sharing philosophies' necessary to under-pin such developments and prevent the possibility of a 'hierarchy of roles' developing.

It is worth mentioning prepared mentor packages at this point. There are a variety of models available which I refer to as:

- *The 'take-away'* ready-made off-the-shelf and just add to your organization or department.
- *The 'Savile Row'* made to measure and tailored to your organization's individual needs.
- *The 'Pick 'n' Mix'* selecting from ready-made models and adapted to your individual preference.

When considering bought in, prepared or tailored mentoring packages there are important questions to consider:

(1) Are they flexible for the organization's needs? Does the programme match the mission, aims, philosophies, value systems, and culture?
(2) How are the mentors' roles and functions perceived? How does this fit with existing support and development roles that already exist in the organisation?
(3) What are the cost implications of buying and then running the programme?
(4) Is programme evaluation included and how does it operate?
(5) Can a sound, cost-effective programme be prepared within the organisation?

Mentor–mentoree preparation and support

This is a developing field at present, with the type, duration of pre-paration and resulting support networks for the mentors appearing as extremely varied. A range of formal programmes exists. This relates to a continuum ranging from those closely aligned to the characteristics of classical mentoring (Hernandez-Piloto Brito, 1992), to the more formal functional structures where contracts are set and mentors assigned and monitored (Anforth, 1992) (see Fig. 3.4).

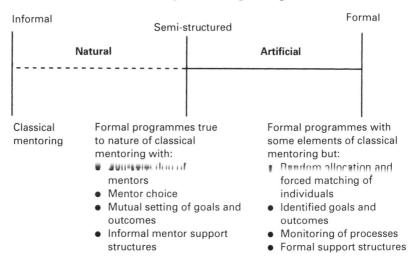

Fig. 3.4   Mentoring: the continuum of informality and formality.

The main contentious issues appear to be those of mentor selection and mentor–mentoree matching.

Mentor selection

As can be seen from the discussions on classical mentoring, what is important is that the mentor is capable of the qualities, characteristics, and skills inherent within an enabling role. The mentor is required to feel competent, confident and committed to taking part. Failures in the past of not building and maintaining relationships probably resulted from forced matching or random allocation of individuals. This was true particularly, for example, in British nursing education, where staff, irrespective of their experience or expertise, were given mentoring responsibilities for a number of students at a time.

The statement 'appropriately qualified and experienced individual' appears to have become a popular way of identifying possible mentors. It is important to identify what is meant by such a broad statement. The term qualified has formal and informal connotations in this context. It may be interpreted to mean that an individual has completed a recognisable training or education programme, or in its broadest sense it may relate to the capabilities of the mentor in terms of the personal qualities that they possess. It is for the programme developers, educators, administrators and managers within a particular setting to clarify what is meant by appropriately qualified and experienced, and state what it is that they require from mentors.

The mentor pool

To assist in making informed selections a mentor pool may be what is needed. A mentor pool is a group of people with appropriate qualities, abilities and experience to take on the rigours and complexities of mentoring. Ideally, this pool should consist of volunteers who are aware of the nature of mentoring (by personal experience or identified criteria), and who are prepared to become committed to a formal programme.

Setting identified criteria and 'trawling' for mentors can take a variety of forms: some programmes have involved marketing techniques (Hernandez-Piloto Brito, 1992); others ask for volunteers, or prospective mentors are chosen/volunteered by their managers. Being chosen or volunteered has potential drawbacks – minimized if consultation and negotiation take place between all involved. Being volunteered for mentor selection particularly increases the risks of toxic mentoring, mismatching of individuals and personality clashes (Palmer, 1986).

Mentor–mentoree matching

This issue will remain contentious until there is sufficient evidence to demonstrate whether freedom to choose mentors or whether forced matching provides the best method for assigning mentorees. Access to a mentor pool allows individuals to make some form of selection, and this process is assisted if the members of the pool prepare brief mentor-biographies of professional and personal experiences. This will identify main interests, work experiences, and the helper functions on offer to a potential mentoree.

Time will need to be set aside within the programme for sessions where the mentors and mentorees can meet. Introductions, the sharing of relevant biographies and setting guidelines for the relationship may need to be facilitated. The informal meetings that arise from the initial discussions can then be arranged by the individuals concerned.

Effective criteria, appropriate selection and time allotted for 'making the match', should ensure that freedom to choose does, indeed, occur. Issues of mentor:mentoree ratios can tax the uninitiated; however, taking into consideration the time, effort, and commitment required, it is suggested that a mentor should not have more than two mentorees at any one time.

It is also important to build workshop sessions into a programme to follow up on any mentors who do not get selected. This may be important with the development of such a new initiative and where mentors are selected by their managers. Until the parameters have been tested and flexibly set, it may be the case that people will be asked to attend a mentor course by managers and administrators in order to gain enabling skills. Rather in the traditional manner of being sent on communication courses to learn how to communicate! It needs to be stressed to all concerned that this is not the aim of mentor programmes.

This should become less of a problem as mentoring becomes a better understood concept and as selection criteria are more adequately addressed. Complementary, enabling programmes can be devised and worked into a framework of continuing education that will feed into appropriate support role programmes to inform other staff who may be involved only indirectly.

The programme

The essence of mentor preparation involves an exploration of the nature of mentoring, the processes, benefits and limitations. Programme aims, strategies, content and outcomes will vary considerably depending on the needs of the organization and personnel. It is important that the programme has clear, well-defined outcomes. It should facilitate:

- An understanding of support within continuing professional development.
- The clarification of new roles and support frameworks.
- Opportunities to enhance enabling skills in relation to the helper functions.
- Feedback on individual performance.
- Opportunities for shared learning.
- Networks of personal support and guidance.
- Understanding of toxic strategies and possible role conflict.
- An understanding of the organization.

Many care workers and professionals in the health field already have preparation containing elements of this type of programme. What needs to be stressed, however, is the need to refocus on certain attitudes and skills to include coaching, instruction and feedback that may not be readily apparent in other continuing education programmes.

It is also crucial to the effectiveness of such a programme that the aims, teaching, facilitating and support strategies should be congruent with the open and enabling philosophy of this type of relationship. It is also important that programme aims or philosophies match those of the organization.

There is no universally agreed length of programme. Some mentor preparation has been included in statutory Teaching and Assessing courses. This usually involves the allotment of two hours or an afternoon to discover the complexities of mentoring. Other programmes have been devised to incorporate a series of workshop days to facilitate a better understanding. Suggestions have been made that a basic training of five days is appropriate with more time for the actual processes (Wright, 1990; Kelly *et al.*, 1991).

Evidence is beginning to emerge regarding the implementation and evaluation of mentoring programmes and formal mentoring approaches based on assigning contract mentors. *The Mentor's Task: Main Activities and Standards* prepared by Oxford Polytechnic (now the Oxford Brookes University) and Oxford Health Authority is documented in Heslop & Lathlean (1991, p. 113).

An investigation into the development and running of an Initial Teacher Training (ITT) course mentor programme is analysed by Corbett & Wright (1993). Their two-year, school-based ITT programme involved asking head teachers to select a teacher to act as a mentor for those on the course. Mentors were offered financial reward and some freeing of their time by one half-day per week supply cover. Certain issues surfaced as the study progressed, these included:

- The crucial role of the head teacher in setting the mentor culture.
- Teacher's development was linked to the development of the mentor.
- Certain groups of individuals appeared better suited to provide the mentor role. These were identified as those new to teaching and those with more experience but with no senior management responsibilities.
- Effective skills and approaches concerned areas of organization, communication, counselling, supporting, monitoring, collaboration and problem solving.
- A willingness to learn, develop and engage in learning were viewed as necessary attributes for mentor selection. Mentors needed to recognize change in their mentorees, and to allow them to establish their own capabilities and responses.
- Mentor training was found to be a restrictive term and mentor development better advised. It should include broad range activities such as attending conferences, manager support, accredited study and informal mentor networks.

Respecting that it is not advisable to generalize from one study, it is interesting to note that these aspects of the analysis are very helpful in going some way towards validating previous deliberations. They also offer evidence for the type of considerations and decisions to be made for those planning similar mentoring schemes.

Supporting the mentor

By providing effective programmes mentors are able to make contact with each other. Depending on the degree of formality of the structured programme on offer, they can build their own networks. Highly experienced individuals of the calibre required to be effective mentors will already, as discussed earlier, have made themselves a niche in the organization.

The need for recognizable and more structured methods of support for mentors has mainly arisen due to the indiscriminate use of this concept in some clinical fields. Support should be negotiable, informal, and the mechanisms developed by the mentors themselves. They can then feel free to identify the issues they wish to explore.

Excessive formal structure with monitoring and feedback reflects traditional rigidity that is inappropriate for this type of enabling relationship or programme. It may deflect some of the intricate interactions from that of the mentor–mentoree partnership and raise concerns regarding the maintenance of confidentiality and mutuality.

Evaluation

Evaluation plays an important part of professional practice and it is an essential element in any new design process. Its importance in constructing formal mentoring programmes is significant because of the lack of empirical evidence and the confusion and contentious nature of the concept (McIntyre, Hagger & Wilkin, 1993). Information obtained from using sound evaluation techniques may aid future developments.

A combination of quantitative and qualitative evaluation approaches are useful to illuminate the complexities of making formal programmes work in practice settings. Such studies should be set within the context of a realistic assessment of the resources available. This is elaborated by Puetz (1992) in her discussion of evaluation and staff development issues. A checklist for designing an evaluation of a programme has been formulated by Murray & Owen (1991, p. 172). In considering the appropriate approaches to be used, it is recommended that both the value to the individual and to the organization should be included in any evaluation deliberations.

Mentoring case studies

These case studies are not intended to be fully representative, but to provide an outline of different types of mentoring relationships. Indeed, in two of the studies presented concerns are raised and mentoring does not appear to have occurred in the richness that is so often reported. Many informal and formal mentoring relationships are positive and develop (through the stages identified previously in this chapter) to become very useful and enabling for all those involved. Presenting these practical applications allows the issues surrounding mentoring to be highlighted and explored.

As you read through the studies you might like to identify relevant issues that you feel are important in relation to what has been discussed in this chapter and your own experiences.

The new community midwife

Chris is a very experienced community midwife in her early 30s. She is keen, quick-thinking and considered by those around her as a good manager, being both well liked and respected by her peers and the women she is responsible for. She enjoys teaching and, 'Seeing those around me settle in, obtain midwifery experience and get on'.

When Pauline, a new midwife joins the district, Chris elects to orientate her and the two of them hit it off immediately. Pauline is a mature woman who has returned to community midwifery, 'After taking time out to have the children'. Despite the obvious age gap Chris senses 'Something of myself' in Pauline's attitudes and responses to her work with the mothers and babies.

They get on well together during Pauline's orientation period with Chris interested in sharing her experience of the busy district. When work load and team commitments allow, the two spend time together discussing their cases and experiences. Pauline is quick to learn, respects Chris's judgement and shows a willingness to become involved in all aspects of midwifery in the district. They remain good working companions and although Pauline always appears eager to meet more often, they manage to meet infrequently because of the changing nature of community midwifery care and their differing shifts. Chris makes time but gradually meeting up together becomes a rare event. Chris is disappointed that the opportunities to share good practice and discuss 'Our ideas for the future of midwifery have become less and less, as we pass like two ships in the night'.

Newly qualified and moving on

Sue is 26 years old and a student midwife. Recently she worked as a staff nurse on a renal surgical ward at the hospital that she trained in. As a third-year student she did well on this particular placement and found she liked and respected the ward Sister, Carol Williams. On qualifying she asked to go back there to staff and 'to learn about looking after patients with renal problems and ward organization'.

Sister Williams was much older than Sue and nearing retirement but had lost none of her keenness for caring for patients and making them comfortable in hospital. She was always the first to arrive on an early shift and the last to leave on a late one, despite having a family and social commitments. As Sue explains, 'She was part of the Old School and I admired her for her personal abilities and nursing skills, she was always willing to share her experiences and spend time with me. During the first year the sound, easy going relationship continued. Sue was quick to learn and Sister Williams, whilst not singling her out from the other team members for extra support, encouraged and spent time with her. Sue felt trusted to 'run things when Sister wasn't there', and she grew in confidence and became more competent in her abilities to handle difficult situations.

Towards the end of the second year, Sue began to get restless as her friends and colleagues discussed different courses and plans for travelling. She shared her thoughts with Sister who had always been ready to listen and counsel in the past. However, it was different this time and 'I soon became aware that she didn't want to know about me moving on or doing my midwifery which is what I had always wanted to do'. Sue went ahead and applied and was accepted for a midwifery programme in the autumn. She was unprepared for Sister's negative response to the news. Despite maintaining a semblance of cordiality whilst working together for the remainder of her notice, Sue and Sister never really spoke again. Sue left the ward without saying goodbye, 'as Sister changed her day off and didn't attend my leaving party'.

Mature and keen to care

Peter is a physiotherapy student. He has had numerous jobs and spent the last few years as an air-traffic controller. He decided to become a physiotherapist after caring for a relation following a road traffic accident. He is one of only three mature students on his course and the only male student. He is enjoying the course and gets on well with his peers although he sometimes gets 'frustrated by their lack of life experience and flippant attitudes to serious concerns'. He is doing well academically and as the course has a formal mentor scheme he is assigned a mentor for his first clinical placement.

Elizabeth is a bright, articulate, eager to teach individual who is younger than Peter. She volunteered for the mentor scheme and enjoys 'The one-to-one relationship with a colleague, teaching and advising them and seeing them develop as they come to terms with what is expected of them as a student and finally a qualified physiotherapist'. Initially Peter and Elizabeth appear to get on well, but gradually Elizabeth becomes aware that Peter does not readily seek her company. He only reluctantly meets with her, when she suggests they get together to discuss his progress in the clinical placements and on the course. Over several months with little progress and tensions on both sides Peter asks his personal tutor if he can change mentors and choose his own this time.

The teacher and mentoring comparisons

Amy is a teacher and she has had 'two significant mentoring relationships', as she puts it, in her career as a teacher. She is currently a faculty head in a department for children with special needs having moved from Expressive Arts recently. When she started as a young teacher she formed a mutually supportive relationship with the head of her department. They got on well, sharing the same views on teaching and had a similar sense of humour. They worked very well together and Amy found that Jan helped her settle in to her new teaching role, as well as helping her to learn about how the school worked. In the early stages of the relationship Amy found that she relied on Jan for her considerable expertise and extensive knowledge. In return Amy would share her ideas and was happy to take on the projects that Jan put her way.

When Jan left to take up a senior teacher's post in a neighbouring community school, it was mutually agreed that Amy would move to the same school as there was a vacant post at a higher incentive allowance. To Amy it seemed 'A sensible option and there was also the possibility of promotion and of course Jan was going too'. After a successful interview, Amy joined the Expressive Arts faculty.

In the new school Amy settled in well and her relationship with Jan 'Continued much as before'. However, after several months Amy became aware that Jan, who initially shared ideas and appeared keen to promote their joint work and projects was changing. In the new setting Jan 'Was now taking my ideas and putting them forward as her own, she even presented a paper at an INSET day that I had written without acknowledging me'. 'I felt I was doing all the hard work, but kept in the background'. Amy attempted to talk this over with Jan with little effect.

Amy left to head a faculty in a new school at the beginning of the new term. She now feels settled and is experiencing a much more positive, working relationship with a deputy head that is supportive and enabling. 'I feel I'm developing in an equal power relationship, able to be me and getting credited with what I do best'. She feels she can be creative, share her ideas and has something to offer her new mentor and faculty.

Classical mentoring: positive returns

Karen was a young occupational therapist when she first joined the faculty of health sciences at a new London university. She had enjoyed the clinical aspects of occupational therapy (OT) but had always been drawn to teaching, 'interested in sharing knowledge and clinical expertise'. She completed a Post Graduate Certificate in Education at the university and then joined the staff, as a lecturer. Karen is an outgoing, affable person who has a keen sense of fun and a deep commitment to her chosen profession.

Following the first year in her lecturing post she remained undecided about a career in higher education and felt 'The loss of my clinical identity, I missed the patients, clients and team work'. She found working with the students rewarding but experienced difficulties in settling into what was a 'Rather traditional department with old-fashioned approaches to teaching and learn-ing at a time when educational methods were advancing'

Karen's attempts at introducing problem-based learning to one of her courses was met with resistance by other members of the department. She was feeling unsettled when a chance meeting with the head of the department, Edwina, altered her perspective. Edwina was a visionary, and extremely capable with an encouraging, honest manner. She did not take herself too seriously despite her position and stature in the OT world. Edwina spoke of the changes and the dilemmas that were occurring as new approaches and methods were considered in OT. She spoke of her commitment to developing education initiatives that would benefit the students, their patients and assist staff to come to terms with the challenges in education and health. This 'Sounded like a blueprint for a better future and I could identify with that', Karen remembers afterwards.

Following their initial meeting, Edwina invited Karen to join a faculty working party to develop a new curriculum. Over a period of time Karen found herself more and more involved in the affairs of the department and taking increasing responsibility for new projects. This led to a more settled feeling and 'A renewed sense of purpose; I felt as if a new, wider world had opened up and that I was very much a part of it'.

The relationship with Edwina was developing positively and Karen found she could discuss issues with her, even 'When I put my foot in it and got things wrong, I was assisted to see the error of my ways without being made to feel insignificant'; 'I could be creative and take some risks, but as time went on, the risks and mistakes reduced as Edwina and I became in tune'. When the principal lecturer's post was advertised Karen felt confident to apply and despite strong external opposition, impressed the panel with her abilities.

Following this senior appointment she found herself working more closely with Edwina, observing her style of management and leadership qualities at first hand. As their relationship developed, and was openly acknowledged as that of classical mentoring, Karen began to specifically choose the assistance she needed: 'At first, I wanted everything Edwina had to offer, it was exciting and stimulating; as time went on, I felt confident to make choices for myself. I asked to be sponsored for a course and I began to know instinctively when I needed counselling or just advice'. With Edwina's support, Karen joined the College of Occupational Therapy as a regional council member. She began to play a part in exploring wider concerns of the profession. 'Edwina opened up a new world to me by asking me to join committees and, ultimately, as our respect and trust grew I began to take her place at certain meetings'. Karen found that they worked out ideas together in a relationship where challenges and tensions could be met head on and strategies devised for success.

After seven years Karen knew it was time to move on: 'I felt capable of taking a leadership role for myself'. Together they explored the possibilities of future job prospects. Karen felt that at the start Edwina was rather reticent at the thought of her moving on: 'She would mention a post, leave the job description on my desk and say"Don't think about it too long"'. Talking over the proposed move together, however, made it more real. Karen's reflections of this period suggest that it was a time of excitement at the prospects of new horizons but sadness as a chapter closed in her working life. 'I felt I was getting ahead now and Edwina admitted that sometimes she felt she was following in my footprints instead of leading the way'.

Finally, after discovering the same post in separate advertisements, Karen successfully applied for the head of school post at a northern university. She is now a nationally respected figure representing OT at the highest levels. Edwina has now retired but Karen and Edwina remain in regular contact and have become firm friends who still like nothing better than getting together to discuss OT issues and the changes that lie ahead.

Case studies: the issues

Sue and Sister Williams built up a good relationship that started when Sue went originally to the ward in the final year of her education programme. They have a mutual interest in their chosen speciality and common commitments to patient care and ward management. What starts for Sue as admiration and role modelling is extended to a more rounded, enabling relationship as Sister gives time to her and shares her clinical expertise. Sue is willing to learn, and with her motivation and interest in the ward she becomes a worthwhile partner in caring for the patients. It is readily apparent that mutual admiration and respect has developed.

Problems occur when Sue wishes to move on. Sister is possessive and not ready to let go. She is nearing retirement and possibly fears the changes that will result when Sue leaves. She has also invested time and effort into the relationship. Careful negotiation and a gradual separation is required in this type of situation. Mentor possessiveness is a more common criticism offered by mentorees in formal mentoring. Feelings of being trapped can occur when the mentoree is submissive and unable to remove themselves from what they see as a claustrophobic situation.

In formal mentoring, making both individuals fully aware of the processes and phases of mentoring can go some way towards preventing this difficulty and allowing endings to be positive. As it is, Sue is unable to resolve the situation. She is unprepared for Sister Williams' distancing behaviour and the relationship ends negatively without the rewards of maintaining contact and friendship.

Pauline is returning to midwifery in the community and although having to face new challenges, she is mature. She may well know her own mind at this time of her life or indeed may not recognize the need for support at this stage. Chris and Pauline are mutually attracted, and work well together. Chris is apparently sending out mentor signals but these are not being picked up by Pauline as she settles into the rigours of busy practice life. Work commitments, lack of regular contact and different shift systems are inhibiting the natural processes of mentoring from taking place.

Although Chris has been helpful in orientating Pauline and assisting her to settle in her new post, there is no time to build on the mutual attraction and respect that has initially occurred. Chris appears ready to mentor and it is highly probable that she will continue to send out signals that will be eventually received when an appropriate individual and right circumstances prevail.

Peter is a mature student. He has been assigned a mentor, in this case a younger female who is keen to help him in his first placement. Peter may be well aware of his needs and we do not know how he has been prepared for the mentoring experience. Sound preparation, with time allotted to get properly acquainted assists potential mentorees to set realistic expectations.

Peter's case also raises issues of cross-gender mentoring and, although not identified here, there are other implications when contract mentoring involves individuals from differing cultures and ethnic groups. Cross-gender mentoring is extensively covered in business and can be associated with sexual liaisons either actual or implied by others who are motivated by favouritism or jealousy. The possibility of sexual tensions and attractions between individuals of different or the same sex should be acknowledged in initial mentor orientation and the outcomes and complications discussed openly.

Risks of personality clashes can occur when mentors are assigned and a mismatch occurs. From the authors' own research and anecdotal evidence, if an assigned mentor is not seen to be meeting the needs of the assigned mentoree, and if there is any dissatisfaction or hostility, then the mentoree will seek a more appropriate individual and set up informal mentoring networks. These often run parallel to those planned and directed by the staff educators. We do not know what preparation

Peter has had or his expectations for this type of relationship, but he draws our attention to issues of the choice in selecting a mentor. It is also important to consider Elizabeth's preparation and experience of mentoring; she may have only been assigned younger or female students previously.

Amy and Jan's case illustrates potential power relationships in mentoring which make evoke reactions and endings similar to those between Sue and Sister Williams. In this situation, Jan with her charisma and winning ways could be seen as enticing the submissive Amy. In negative terms, Jan is using her to further her own development and career. Mutuality has ceased and the power balance has shifted towards that of meeting the needs of a powerful, controlling mentor.

Amy has changed jobs and the focus has moved from her own needs and development to that of maintaining Jan's credibility. This study presents us with an example of the 'queen bee/worker bee syndrome': if one party remains submissive and readily supplies the 'queen bee' the two can advance through the hierarchy together until circumstances cause them to fall out or drift apart. In this example, Amy is able to recognize what is happening and is very capable in acting quickly to get herself out of the situation. She is then able to commence a new relationship with the deputy head in the new school. This relationship is much more aligned to that of true classical mentoring. Amy experiences none of the toxicity of the previous encounter and is able to feel confident in sharing in more collaborative surroundings.

The last case demonstrates the positive aspects of classical mentoring in terms of the natural nature of the collaboration – the mutual rewards and the longevity as the two individuals start to trust, share and respect each other. Similar in essence to the supportive and enabling relationship that Amy (in the previous case) has begun at her new school. Karen's commitment and need for change is recognized by her senior colleague. A relationship develops that assists Karen to sort out her feelings about her career, to become involved in departmental initiatives and to rehearse areas of learning that facilitates an awareness of her own abilities.

In the early stages of the relationship Karen notes the need for any type of support and is not discerning in selecting what she requires. However, as the mutual trust, honest communication and respect builds, she becomes more confident to choose the assistance she requires. Karen is well aware of the risks she takes and the development that occurs. The personal guidance offered is such that she maintains her self-esteem and confidence, as well as being encouraged to learn from less positive events. Karen is able to develop her own professional identity constructively, eventually leading to her taking a significant leadership role. Edwina, in her retirement, can feel satisfied that she played a part in Karen's success and that she has left OT in capable hands.

These cases have demonstrated a range of issues. You will have identified others within the examples given and from consideration of your own experiences. It is only by illuminating mentoring in all its many forms and by understanding how it works in practice, that we will be able to provide adequate programmes of preparation in the future. A clearer understanding will go some way towards removing the scepticism and negative effects that may arise from using the concept inappropriately and with little thought. Effective programmes and increased knowledge will also assist in encouraging those qualified practitioners wanting to become mentors to view mentoring as a recognition of their qualities, approachability and professionalism, and not as a 'right'.

References

Anforth, P. (1992) Mentors, not assessors. *Nurse Education Today*, **12** (4), 299–302.

Armitage, P. & Burnard, P. (1991) Mentors or Preceptors? Narrowing the theory–practice gap. *Nurse Education Today*, **11** (3), 225–9.

Ashton, P. & Richardson. G. (1992) Preceptorship and PREPP. *British Journal of Nursing*, **1** (3), 143–6.

Ball, C. (1992) The Learning Society. *Royal Society of Arts Journal*, May, 380–94.

Barlow, S. (1991) Impossible dream. *Nursing Times*, 87 (1) 53–4.

Blotnick, S. R. (1984) With friends like these. *Savvy*, **10**, 45–52.

Burnard, P. (1988) Self-evaluation methods in nurse education. *Nurse Education Today*, **8** (4), 229–33.

Calkins, E.V., Arnold, L.M. & Willoughby, T.L. (1987) Perceptions of the role of a faculty supervisor or 'mentor' at two medical schools. *Assessment and Evaluation in Higher Education*, **12** (3) 202–8

Campbell-Heider, N. (1986) Do nurses need mentors? *IMAGE: Journal of Nursing Scholarship*, **18** (3) 110–13.

Cantor, L.M. & Roberts, I.F. (1986) *Further Education Today: A Critical Review.* (3rd edition) Routledge Kegan Paul, London.

Clutterbuck, D. (1985) *Everybody Needs A Mentor – How To Further Talent Within An Organisation.* The Institute of Personnel Management, London.

Collins, E.G.C. & Scott, P. (1978) Everybody who makes it has a mentor. *Harvard Business Review*. July/August, 89–102.

Cooper, M.D. (1990) Mentorship: the key to the future of professionalism in nursing. *Journal of Perinatal and Neonatal Nursing*, **4** (3), 71–77.

Corbett, P. & Wright, D. (1993) Issues in the selection and training of mentors for school-based primary teaching training, in *Mentoring: Perspectives on School-based Teacher Education*, McIntyre, D., Hagger, H. and Wilkin, M.), pp. 220–33. Kogan Page, London.

Darling, L.A.W. (1984) What do nurses want in a mentor? *Journal of Nursing Administration*, **14** (10), 42–44.

Darling, L.A.W. (1986) What to do about toxic mentors. *Nurse Educator*, **11** (2), 29–30.

DFE, (1992) *Initial Teacher Training (Secondary Phase)*, (Circular 9/92). Department for Education, London.

ENB, (1987) *Institutional and Course Approval/Reapproval Process, Information Required – Criteria and Guidelines*, 1987/28/MAT; English National Board, London.

ENB, (1988) *Institutional and Course Approval/Reapproval Process, Information Required – Criteria and Guidelines*, 1988/39/APS. English National Board, London.

Eng, S.P. (1986) Mentoring in principalship education, in Murray, M. with Owen, M.A. (eds) *Beyond the Myths and Magic of Mentoring: How to Facilitate an Effective Mentor Program*. Jossey-Bass, Oxford.

Fagan, M.M. & Walter, G. (1982) Mentoring among teachers. *Journal of Education Research*, **76** (2), 113–18.

Fields, W.L. (1991) Mentoring in Nursing: a historical approach. *Nursing Outlook*, Nov/Dec, 257–61.

George, P. & Kummerow, J. (1981 Mentoring for career women. *Training*, **18** (2), 44; 46–9.

Hagerty, B. (1986) A second look at mentors. *Nursing Outlook* 34 (1) 16–19; 24.

Hamilton, M.S. (1981) Mentorhood, a key to nursing leadership. *Nursing Leadership*, **4** (1) 4–13.

Handy, C. (1985) *Understanding Organisations*. Penguin Business, Harmondsworth.

Hardy, L.K. (1984) The emergence of nurse leaders: In case of, in spite of, not because of. *International Nursing Review*, **31** (1), 11–15.

Hawkins, J.W. & Thibodeau, J.A. (1989) *The Nurse Practitioner and Clinical Nurse Specialist. Current Practice Issues* (2nd Edn). The Tiresias Press Inc., New York.

Hawkins, P. & Shohet, R. (1989) *Supervision in the Helping Professions*. The Open University, Milton Keynes.

Hernandez/Piloto Brito, H. (1992) Nurses in action: An innovative approach to mentoring. *Journal of Nursing Administration*, **22** (5), 23–8.

Heslop, A. Lathlean, J. (1991 Teaching and Learning. In *Becoming a Staff Nurse – A Guide to the Role of the Newly Registered Nurse* (Ed. by J. Lathlean & J. Corner). Prentice Hall, London.

HMSO, (1972) *Teacher Education and Training*. (The James Report). Her Majesty's Stationery Office, London.

Holt, R. (1982). An alternative to mentorship. *Adult Education,* (**55**) 2, 152–6.

Hunt, D. & Michael, C. (1983) Mentorship. A career training in development tool. *Academy of Management Review,* **3**, 475–85.

James Committee (1972) *Teacher Education and Training (The James Report).* HMSO, London.

Kelly, K.J. (1992) *Nursing Staff Development: Current Competence, Future Focus.* J.B. Lippincott Company, Philadelphia.

Kelly, M., Beck, T. & Thomas, J. (1991) More than a supporting act. *The Times Educational Supplement,* November 8.

Klopf, G.J. & Harrison, J. (1981) Moving up the career ladder: the case of mentors. *Principal,* **61**, 41–3.

Knowles, M.S. (1984) *Andragogy in Action: Applying Modern Principles of Adult Learning,* Jossey-Bass, San Francisco.

Lathlean, J. & Corner, J. (1991) *Becoming a Staff Nurse – A Guide to the Role of the Newly Registered Nurse.* Prentice Hall International, Hemel Hempstead.

Levinson, D.J., Darrow, C.N., Klein, D.B., Levinson, M.H. & McKee, B. (1978) *The Seasons of a Man's Life.* Knopf, New York.

Kay, K.M., Meleis, A.I. & Winstead-Fry, P. (1982) Mentorship for scholarliness, opportunities and dilemmas. *Nursing Outlook,* **30**, 22–8.

McIntyre, D., Hagger, H. & Wilkin, M. (1993) *Mentoring: Perspectives on School-Based Teacher Education.* Kogan Page, London.

Merriam, S. (1983) Mentors and protégés: a critical review of the literature. *Adult Education Quarterly,* **33** (3), 161– 73.

Monaghan, J. & Lunt, N. (1992) Mentoring: person, process, practice and problems. *The British Journal of Educational Studies,* **XXXX** (3), 239–47.

Morle, K.M.F. (1990) Mentorship, is it a case of the emperor's new clothes or a rose by any other name. *Nurse Education Today,* **10** (1), 66–9.

Muller, S. (1984) Physicians for the twenty-first century: report of the project panel on general professional education of the physician's preparation for medicine. *Journal of Medical Education,* **59**, p. 2.

Murray, M. & Owen, M.A. (1991) *Beyond the Myths and Magic of Mentoring: How to Facilitate an Effective Mentor Program.* Jossey-Bass, Oxford.

Nixon, N. & Fenwick, A. (1993) *Developing Students' Subject Area Knowledge and Skills in the Work Place.* Working group briefing paper. The Open University, London.

Palmer, E.A. (1986) *Evaluation Notes II for Enrolled Nurse Conversion.* Unpublished project report, St. Mary's School of Nursing, London.

Palmer, E.A. (1987) *The Nature of the Mentor Relationship in Nurse Education: A Study to Introduce the Mentor. Unpublished thesis, South Bank Polytechnic, London.*

Palmer, E.A. (1992) *The Role of the Mentor in Critical Care.* Conference Paper, 7th Annual Conference, The British Association of Critical Care Nurses, Manchester University.

Parsons, S.F. (1993) Feminist challenges to curriculum design, in Thorpe, M., Edwards, R. & Hanson, A. (eds) *Culture and Processes of Adult Learning.* Routledge, The Open University, London.

Pratt, J.W. (1989) Towards a philosophy of physiotherapy. *Physiotherapy,* **75** (2), 114–20.

Puetz, B.E. (1992) Evaluation: essential skill for the staff development specialists, in Kelly, K.J. (ed) *Nursing Staff Development: Current Competence, Future Focus. J.B. Lippincott & Co., Philadelphia.*

Puetz, B.E. (1985) Learn the ropes from a mentor. *Nursing Success Today,* **2** (6), 11–13.

Raichura, L. & Riley, M. (1985) Introducing nurse preceptors, *Nursing Times* Nov. 20, 40–42.

Roche, G.R. (1979) Much ado about mentors. *Harvard Business Review,* **56**, 14–18. Jan/Feb.

Rogers, C.R. (1983) *Freedom to Learn for the Eighties.* Charles E. Merrill & Co., Columbus, Ohio.

Safire, W. (1980) On language, *New York Times Magazine,* Nov., 1980 reported to George, P. & Kummerow, J. Mentoring for career women, *Training,* **18** (2), 44; 46–9.

Sheehy, G. (1976) The mentor connection and the secret link in the successful woman's life. *New York Magazine,* **8**, 33–9.

Shapiro, E.C., Haseltine, F. & Rowe, M. (1978) Moving up: role models, mentors and the patron system. *Sloan Management Review,* **19**, 51–8.

UKCC (1990) *The Report of the Post-Registration Education and Practice Project,* United Kingdom Central Council, 183–201.

Vance, C.N. (1979) Women leaders: modern-day heroines or societal deviants? *IMAGE: Journal of Nursing Scholarship,* **11** (2), 40–1.

Vance, C.N. (1982) The mentor connection. *The Journal of Nursing Administration,* **12** (4), 7–13.

Weil, S. (1992) Learning to change, in *Managing Fundamental Change: Shaping New Purposes and Roles in Public Services.* Report of a one day conference organized by the Office for Public Management. June, 1992.

Wheatley, M. & Hirsch, M.S. (1984) Five ways to leave your mentor. *MS Magazine,* Sept. 106–8.

Wright, C.M. (1990) An innovation in a diploma programme: the future potential of mentorship in nursing. *Nurse Education Today,* **10** (5), 355–9.

Zaleznik, A. (1977) Manager leaders: are they different? *Harvard Business Review,* **55** (3), 67–78.

Zey, M.G. (1984) *The Mentor Connection.* Dow Jones Irwin, Homewood, Illinois.

Recommended reading

Clawson, J.C. & Kram, M.E. (1984) Managing cross-gender mentoring. *Business Horizons,* **27**, 22–32.

Hardy, L.K. (1990) The path to knowledge – personal reflections. *Nurse Education Today,* **10**, 325–32.

Kramer, M. (1968) Role models, role conceptions, and role deprivation. *Nursing Research,* **17** (2), 115–20.

Useful references for:

Conceptual deliberations

Anderson, E. & Shanon, A. (1988) Towards a conceptualization of mentoring. *Journal of Teacher Education*, **39** (1), 38–42

Palmer, A. (1987) *The Nature of the Mentor Relationship in Nurse Education: A Study to Introduce the Mentor*, Unpublished thesis, South Bank Polytechnic, London.

Puetz, B.E. (1985) Learn the ropes from a mentor. *Nursing Success Today*, **2** (6), 11–13.

Yoder, L. (1990) Mentoring: a concept analysis. *Nursing Administration Quarterly*, **15** (1), 9–19.

Mentor qualities and characteristics

Clutterbuck, D. (1985) Everybody needs a mentor – how to further talent within an organization. *The Institute of Personnel Management*, London.

George, P. & Kummerow, J. (1981) Mentoring for career women, *Training*, **18** (2), 44; 46–9.

May, K.M., Meleis, A.I. & Winstead-Fry, P. (1982) Mentorship for scholarliness: opportunities and dilemmas. *Nursing Outlook*, **30** (1), 22–8.

Zey, M.G. (1984) *The Mentor Connection*. Dow Jones Irwin, Homewood, Illinois.

Formal programmes

Hernandez-Piloto Brito, H. (1992) Nurses in action: an innovative approach to mentoring. *Journal of Nursing Administration*, 22 (5), 23–8.

Monaghan, J. & Lunt, N. (1992) Mentoring: person, process, practice and problems. *British Journal of Educational Studies*, **XXXX** (3), 239–47.

Murray, M. & Owen, M.A. (1991) *Beyond the Myths and Magic of Mentoring: How to Facilitate an Effective Mentor Program*. Jossey-Bass, Oxford.

Hagerty, B. (1986) A second look at mentors. *Nursing Outlook*, **34** (1), 16–19; 24.

Chapter 4
Preceptor Support Systems

The search for adequate definitions and guidance on the teaching and support roles offered to nursing staff has sometimes been hampered by the apparent overlap between these roles. As we have seen, the differences need to be clarified in order to make the preparation for both roles appropriate to the demands made on them.

Unfortunately, the myths and misunderstandings which have grown up around both mentoring and preceptorship have made the terms virtually interchangeable, and as a result much of what can be achieved by preceptorship has been unclear.

This chapter hopes to remedy this, and to clarify what is both special and different about the preceptor role, and to provide the background information necessary to introduce a preceptorship system into the workplace.

The potential for preceptorship across the health care professions is wide and varied. Much of what is needed in terms of personnel, administrative systems and specialist expertise already exists in the workplace, both in acute and community service settings. Preceptorship only requires a change of emphasis and a willingness to adopt that change if it is to be successful in harnessing the potential resources available. But what exactly is preceptorship and how can it be operationalized?

What is preceptorship?

Preceptorship is a form of educational relationship which is intended to provide newly qualified (or returning) professionals with three things:

(1) Access to an experienced and competent role model.
(2) A means by which to build a supportive one-to-one teaching and learning relationship.
(3) A smooth transition from learner to accountable practitioner.

As such, its strengths lie in enabling practitioners to develop their knowledge and skills in an atmosphere of trust, with colleagues who have experienced for themselves, and who have been prepared for, and understand, the challenges confronting the beginning practitioner.

The word 'precept' is derived from the Latin *praeceptum*, meaning order, maxim, or authoritative command; one of the practical rules of an art. A 'praeceptor' is described as a teacher, tutor or instructor: as one who heads a 'praeceptory', i.e. 'a subordinate community of Knights Templars' dating from the fifteenth century (SOED).

Its evolution in nursing appears to have developed in the United States in the 1970s, when the need for an early socialization phase in nursing became evident in American nursing schools. Kramer (1974) observed that moving from the protected world of the student into the reality of everyday practice presented traumatic and difficult choices for new staff, requiring them to synthesize what they had learned and apply it, often at speed, and with consequences which they were expected to anticipate and make allowances for in reaching clinical decisions.

According to Magill *et al.* (1986) educational relationships tend to take one of four forms along a continuum. They may be:

- *Didactic relationships* which emphasize the transfer of information from teacher to learner.
- *Supervisory relationships* which emphasize close direction of the learner by the teacher.
- *Collaborative relationships* which emphasize responsibility shared by the teacher.
- *Consultative relationships* which emphasize teacher response to narrowly defined requests from learners.

Although these authors are describing such roles in relation to medical education, they stress the need for all educational relationships to be empirically researched in order for such concepts to be properly validated and accepted in the clinical setting (Magill, France & Munning, 1986).

What makes preceptorship special?

The distinguishing characteristic which sets apart preceptorship from other models of continuing education is that it enjoys a central element of support: support between colleagues, support for learning, and support for the person who is undergoing the critical developmental transition phases in his or her career.

In traditional modes, teaching may be considered active and learning relatively passive. Because preceptorship is based on a one-to-one method of teaching and learning, the content and direction of which is negotiated between preceptor partners, it is ideally placed to provide a structure for the educational process which is holistic and which allows for the individual personalities, situations and learning styles of both preceptor and 'preceptee'.

Preceptorship is an attempt to redefine the process of learning in a way which emphasizes the individuality of the learner and the dynamics of learning as interactive and unpredictable.

It allows us to plan for learning, and yet at the same time to respond to those 'teachable moments' which arise from time to time, often without warning, and which can yield valuable lessons and insight into the care we are learning to give.

If we wanted to, we could adopt preceptorship as the predominant form of continuing learning for all beginning professionals in health care, but to do this successfully requires the commitment of experienced staff to participate fully in the role, and wider recognition of the validity of learning experienced in day-to-day practice.

With increasing attention being given to accreditation of prior experiential learning, the time may be ripe to develop such work-based concepts further, and to build them into flexible opportunities for accruing recognized credits in tandem with other more established forms of continuing learning, such as open learning, self-study modules, day release and study secondments, evening classes and in-service training days. With a little adaptation and a good deal of co-operation, preceptorship could become the model for all continuing professional education, beginning the moment a person qualifies, and providing an ethos and an enthusiasm for learning that carries on throughout working life.

Preceptorship in nursing

Preceptorships in nursing are well established in North America, but existing definitions of the concept can be inaccurate and misleading for use in the UK because of differences in the educational preparation of nurses in the USA and Canada.

Shamian & Inhaber (1985), for example, write that the nursing profession has adapted and modified the traditional tutor–instructor role of preceptor to describe:

> 'a unit based nurse who carries out one to one teaching of new employees or nursing students, in addition to her regular unit duties'.

> (Shamian & Inhaber, 1985, p. 79)

In British terms, however, the preceptor role is intended for use as a mechanism for structuring *continuing* education in nursing, and we need to make clear that the relationship is one of peers and partners, rather than qualified member of staff and student/learner.

Unlike the USA, the preceptor relationship in the UK refers to a relationship between two qualified practitioners, both of whom are accountable for their practice (UKCC, 1993).

The British nurse preceptor will share a great deal in common with her North American colleague, as we shall see later in this chapter, but for purely pragmatic reasons which have been historically determined in the UK, the British nurse preceptor could be more accurately defined or described as:

'... a qualified and experienced first-level nurse, midwife or health visitor who has agreed to work in partnership with a (newly) registered practitioner colleague in order to assist and support them in the process of learning and adaptation to his or her new role'.

(Morton-Cooper, 1993)

As such, the role will focus on the learning and socialization needs of the newly registered practitioner and those returning to practice after a substantial break in service.

Lessons to be learned from the North American literature

In a very pragmatic outline of what has happened to nursing education in the last 30 years, Backenstose (1983) writes that clinically based models of teaching and learning in nursing are far from new.

In Florence Nightingale's day, nurses were taught at the bedside by a more experienced nurse, and expected to model their own performance accordingly. The first literal 'preceptors' were actually doctors: they wrote the first nursing textbooks and provided the theoretical input by way of clinical lectures and practical demonstrations. Trained nurses provided experience of 'hands on' nursing under strict supervision both on the wards and in patients' homes.

It was only as nursing education moved to the academic setting in pursuit of professional growth that the 'service–education bond' began to break down. With the development of separate colleges of nursing, tutors acquired higher level positions than those in the service, and therefore widened the gulf between service and education, leading to the now familiarly termed 'service–education divide', or what has been described as 'the theory–practice gap'.

Consequently, nursing students came to be taught didactically and clinically by non-practising nurse educators. The re-introduction of preceptors became necessary in the 1970s when it was realized that nursing could not be taught in isolation from practice, and the orientation of nurses to their work role and the realities of practical nursing had become a priority (Backenstose, 1983, p. 9).

Douville has described preceptorship in the USA as a modified apprenticeship learning system, and as a method of learning that has many advantages because it recognizes nursing education's fundamental need for quality education in both clinical and academic settings:

> 'The preceptor and student, through mutual discussion and agreement on set objectives and goals, enter into a partnership each with different and distinct responsibilities but each with the same commitment – to work towards the established goals. Thus the traditional student–teacher relationship is transcended, and an interaction emerges that is marked more by unity than disparity'.

> (Douville, 1983, p. 123)

The idea of preceptorship emerging in nursing as an opportunity to develop a shared value system is evident elsewhere in the literature, primarily in response to the problems experienced by staff over 'value conflicts'.

Nursing's 'troubled sponsorship'

In a study which looked at problems associated with the new nurse's work entry Benner & Benner (1979) identified some of the major barriers that new nurses experienced in trying to adapt to their new work roles. These centred around perceived value conflicts between the newly graduated nurse and her employers, and around a serious mismatch of expectations regarding the anticipated competence and performance of the new employee (Benner & Benner, 1979).

When interviewed about their expected levels of competency, new graduates expressed the highest expectations; nurse educators on the other hand had lower expectations, and expected new nurses to need considerably more supervision than they themselves had envisaged. Nursing service personnel had the lowest expectations of all. All three groups perceived wide gaps between the ideal (in terms of performance) and reality.

The authors concluded that the discrepancy in their views was sufficient to cause considerable conflict and misinterpretation between them in a work setting, and lead to *negative stereotyping* of the new nurses' abilities. New nurses were expected by their service colleagues to demonstrate skills akin to that of a nursing auxiliary, rather than a fully fledged practitioner.

The new employees were therefore frustrated at times by the lack of knowledge and understanding shown to them by colleagues, and tended to respond in one of two ways: either under-performing (and therefore making the service nurses' perceptions of them a self-fulfilling pro-phecy), or becoming disillusioned with practice, experiencing feelings of disillusionment and antagonism towards colleagues, and perhaps leaving the clinical environment altogether in protest (Benner & Benner, 1979).

The underlying value conflict – or lack of shared values – led to a feeling of dissonance and a further, cyclical negative stereotyping (e.g. 'these new nurses think they know it all'; 'the trained staff seem to have forgotten everything they learned at college', and so on). The need to resolve such a conflict is the reason given as to why 'sponsorship' in the form of support roles has become necessary for nursing.

Benner's more recent interpretation of preceptorship (Benner, 1984) is still true to her original ethos of resolving the troubled sponsorship experienced between new and established nursing staff, and is about encouraging colleagueship among peers; allowing new nurses to gain insight into where divergence from textbook learning about nursing (or 'paradigm cases') is necessary and helpful. She warns that negative stereotyping or blanket appraisal of beginning nurses is based on the normal tendency to give blanket or global appraisals, so that if new nurses are found lacking in one area, they are considered deficient in all other areas.

Nurse managers seem to be especially inclined toward this kind of generalization by significantly underestimating the new nurses' capabilities:

> 'These findings suggest that nurse managers might do well to adjust and balance their negative appraisals in order to create a climate of success. The manager's perception may be distorted by exposure only to problems, with little opportunities to observe success, so the manager may need to deliberately seek out positive examples to balance the picture. It is easier to succeed in a climate where acceptance and expectations of success are the rule rather than the exception'.

(Benner, 1984, p. 190)

A review of the US literature

In a very helpful review of some 21 papers on preceptorship Shamian & Inhaber (1985) remark that the removal of nursing schools from hospital facilities in the US has made high quality initial hospital orientation for new employees vital, particularly for new nurse graduates. They also cite early 'burnout' and lack of satisfaction in new employees as a reason for improving their integration and socialization into new jobs.

The move to provide programmes through which students were assisted in making adjustments from theory to practice met with an enthusiastic response:

> 'The concept of decentralized teaching makes for a non-stressful environment where positive feedback and learning are supported and encouraged... Integration of the new employee into the unit is facilitated by someone who is close to the scene of the activity, and there is good reason to believe that a peer relationship is able to effect the required learning'.

> (Shamian & Inhaber, 1985, pp. 80–81)

They claim that extensive utilization of the preceptorship model has been very successful in meeting the aims of integration for both colleges and hospitals, and conclude from the literature that the core responsibilities of the preceptor should be:

(1) Orientation of preceptees to the unit.
(2) Socialization of preceptees to the unit.
(3) Teaching, observation and evaluation of preceptees.
(4) Assisting in the establishment of objectives and priorities during orientation or internship
(5) Communicating with superiors regarding the progress of preceptees.

> (Shamian & Inhaber, 1985, p. 82)

Prerequisites for selection as a preceptor are offered as years of experience, appropriate leadership skills, communication skills, decision-making ability, and an interest in professional growth, presumably their own and their prospective preceptees.

Hitchings (1989) suggests the introduction of preceptorships as an appropriate response to nursing shortages, saying that such models meet the 'intense, often individual, learning needs of the nurse orientee, and strengthen the educational fabric of the institution' (Hitchings, 1989,

p. 256). She lists the benefits to the employing institution as improvements in staff satisfaction and morale, cost effectiveness, recruitment and retention, and improved quality of care.

Cruz & Riley (1984) stress the mutuality and flexibility offered by preceptorships in that they are helpful for assisting both parties in updating knowledge and skills, providing a fresh perspective on the work environment, increasing participants' self-esteem, and decreasing the education–service gap. They say that in an era of increasing medical technology and shifting demands for nursing skills, nursing is besieged by doubts about its professionalism, basic competence and adaptability:

'The need for a sense of kinship and respect between and among nurses is greater than ever. We feel preceptorships offer a unique way of experiencing kinship while reaping many other rewards.

(Cruz & Riley, 1984, p. 55)

They also point out the advantage of being able to negotiate hours and schedules between the preceptor and preceptee, so that learning isn't fixed immutably to set times and limited opportunities.

Qualities looked for in a preceptor by Parsons *et al.* (1985) were:

- Interest in the development of the staff nurse's skills.
- Leadership and teaching abilities.
- Ability to role model.
- Ability to 'utilize the nursing process and clinical excellence in her area of practice'.

(Parsons, 1985, p. 19)

Others feel that the best use of preceptorship is the opportunity it provides to help learners to become self-directed in their learning. Because the preceptor is a part of the agency, they therefore constitute a realistic role model, rather than the idealized version beheld in nursing school (Dobbie *et al.*, 1982).

These authors envisage the preceptor's responsibilities as those of developing a plan of action that meets the student's personal and course objectives within the realities of the practice setting; of making sure that such a plan is progressive, and allows for a gradual move from a participant–observer stance to that of independent practitioner; and of helping the student to choose which activities will actually assist learning.

Preceptors would also teach, supervise and consult with the student throughout the preceptorship, and participate in the evaluation of the student's performance as designated in any pre-agreed learning contract.

Preceptorship's use as a reward or 'positive reinforcer' of nursing work is also considered by Turnbull (1983), who claims that identifying and developing such positive reinforcers is the key to organizational effectiveness.

Limon *et al.*, (1982) have some salient warnings for service managers and individual practitioners, however, when it comes to the matter of legal accountability.

They warn that perceptions of how accountable the preceptor is in terms of the work carried out by the preceptee should be clarified before any contractual arrangements are finalized between the college arranging the preceptorship and the unit offering the experience.

The need to discuss this aspect with preceptors and preceptees is also extremely important in the British context. In the USA a bona fide as yet unqualified student as well as a newly graduated nurse can be the preceptee, and the legal situation is obviously somewhat different between those of qualified and unqualified status.

In Britain it is proposed that newly qualified staff nurses acting as preceptees will remain accountable for their own actions, however, and it will therefore be interesting to see whether the legal responsibilities of the preceptor to supervise the preceptee (and presumably not misdirect them) are properly explored before any test case or legal action emerges as a consequence of a preceptor giving an ill-judged instruction or direction to the preceptee.

The responsibility for anticipating such a critical dilemma is, of course, the UKCC's, which has its own statutory duty to maintain and improve standards of practice and to protect the public from unsafe practitioners acting in a nursing, midwifery or health visiting capacity.

The question is not simply whether the preceptor abides by the terms of the UKCC Code of Professional Conduct (1992), but whether in fact the preceptor has an additional duty of care to the preceptee as a 'novice' practitioner, and could therefore be described as having greater accountability than her potentially unwitting and less experienced colleague.

Applications of preceptorship within the US nursing curriculum

In the USA the principles of preceptorship have been applied in a number of different ways. Sometimes the preceptor concept is integrated into core courses in the pre-qualifying curriculum, or offered to students as electives in the later part of their initial education. They can also be offered after qualification.

Preceptorships allow the assignment of increasingly complex patients and groups of patients to students in a controlled learning environment (Zerbe *et al.*, 1991). However, these authors point out that while the advantages of preceptorship are widely recognized in the USA, Canada, and Australia, there is as yet little consensus as to the specific organization of preceptor programs and their placement within the curriculum.

Zerbe *et al.*, recommend a three- tiered approach to preceptorship, known as a 'preceptor–student tryad', whereby a third person, known as a 'faculty instructor' (normally faculty- or college-based and 'masters-prepared'), supervises the 'preceptor–student dyad' or partnership

They advocate the use of such instructors because of the need to provide a resource for the preceptor:

> 'The clinical instructor is available for problem-solving and assists with bedside teaching. [He or she also] relays information about course content and objectives to the preceptors, helping them to feel involved with the didactic portion of the course'.

> (Zerbe *et al.*, 1991, p. 20)

One of the major problems when assessing the potential success of transferring a similar model of preceptorship to the British nursing system is that the distinction between student preceptees and staff nurse preceptees becomes evermore critical.

Whereas in the USA students are invariably following a course curriculum with all the curriculum planning, teaching and learning support that such a course entails, what we are intending to do in Britain is to leave the negotiation of teaching and learning methods (in terms of process and content) to the individuals themselves.

While it is possible to provide some generic back-up and introduction in the provision of preceptor preparation programmes and continuing support to preceptors, the time suggested for such programmes in the UK only extends to two days, (UKCC, 1993). The very fact that implementation was envisaged within a very short timescale suggests that Council did not consider or recognize fully in their deliberations how extensive effective preceptor preparation might have to be.

Student preceptees in the Zerbe study said that they often felt uncomfortable with the diversity of learning opportunities and requirements offered by preceptorship, and that they would prefer more standardization of preparation, written assignments, conferences and evaluations. This raises the issue of the ways in which the process and outcomes of the preceptor relationship should be documented in clinical practice. Who will exert control over the dynamics of the one-to-one relationship, and who will help to overcome any problems experienced between the preceptor and preceptee?

Chickerella & Lutz (1981) see 'professional nurturance' as one outcome of successful preceptoring, although they tend to view the preceptor as a facilitator of learning that has originally been laid down by faculty (or the college, in UK terminology). Supervision of the relationship in the USA has therefore primarily been the responsibility of the college, in collaboration and agreement with the service institution.

The attributes of an effective preceptor

Lewis (1986) writes that

> [many] 'forlorn students have reported to their peers and instructors that their preceptorship experience was a disaster, despite the fact that their nurses "really knew their stuff".'

> (Lewis, 1986, p. 18)

Although attributes such as experience in the proposed clinical area were considered important, the possession of sound and empathetic communications skills came top of many students' lists. Honesty, perceptiveness, ability to feed back on performance in a tactful and understanding way were considered extremely important – as was the preceptor's ability to demonstrate genuine caring for her patients' well-being. Being able to demonstrate the organizational and time management of looking after several patients at once was also a quality sought by students, who often floundered when trying to constantly reorganize their priorities for care.

Piemme *et al.* (1987) have devised a list of common characteristics of the 'ideal preceptor', although it is not clear from their work exactly how they arrived at such a list.

The list of qualities of the ideal preceptor includes patience, enthusiasm, knowledge, (of *what* is not stipulated!), they must be well-organized, have a positive attitude, be non-threatening, non-judgemental, flexible, open-minded, objective, have a sense of humour, be mature, have mastered clinical skills, be assertive, act as an advocate for the learner, be able to use resources, be self-confident (while recognizing their own weaknesses), be responsible, professional and respected by their peers (Piemme *et al.*, 1987). They also insist that it is crucial for both preceptors and preceptees to understand the ways in which adults learn.

Expectations of the preceptor relationship

When the preceptor model was introduced in the USA in the 1970s its principal function appears to have been to help staff to manage the transition from new nurse to competent practitioner more expertly, and to dilute the perceived effects of 'reality shock' in the transition of nursing students who were educated in the primarily college setting to that of clinical practice.

This is best expressed in the seminal work of Kramer (1974), who devised a mechanism for dealing with this — a process she described as 'anticipatory socialization'. By providing an effective anticipatory transition phase in students' careers, the argument was that reality shock would be weakened, and integration with reality made more successful. The concept of preceptorship was thus reborn in an attempt to socialize new graduates in the USA into the world of work.

Despite the optimistic claims made for re-socialization via preceptorship (e.g. Clayton *et al.*, 1989; Jairath *et al.*, 1991; Laschinger *et al.*, 1992) Myrick (1988) cites several studies that indicate that there is no significant difference in the clinical performance of those nurses who have been preceptored from those who haven't (e.g. Huber, 1981).

Any evaluation of preceptorship's success is dependent on whether we see the role primarily as a means of helping individuals to adapt and conform to their work roles, as a mechanism for supervising and enhancing nursing performance, or primarily as a support role intended to ease the transition to clinical work with a view to reducing stress on new staff and promoting good employee relationships in the clinical environment. Different studies appear to evaluate the relationship either solely on performance or as an amalgam of all approaches.

The difficulty with measuring preceptorship solely in terms of nursing performance is the question of whose criteria are used to measure that performance: those of the college, the employer, or the statutory bodies for re-licensing of the practitioner?

It could be argued that the criteria used for measurement need to be standardized, or different units will apply criteria haphazardly, and any results will then have difficulty being interpreted accurately by a future prospective employer.

The question this raises is crucial. What do we expect preceptorship to do exactly? We need to clarify our intentions in order to plan and prepare people effectively for the relationship, and to determine outcomes which can be measured so that it can be properly evaluated from the perspectives of role development and continuing nurse education.

Myrick (1988) advocates caution in trusting all to preceptorship, warning against the danger of 'warm body syndrome', which could be interpreted as the temptation to thrust responsibility for any shortfall in pre-registration education on to practising nurses, without fully considering the underlying implications for initial education:

'The "warm body syndrome" frequently prevails in that any nurse who wishes to be a preceptor is acceptable regardless of educational background, experience, or teaching ability. When used in this context, the basic preceptorship premise of facilitating student learning in the clinical setting is obscured'.

(Myrick, 1988, p. 137)

Myrick insists that preceptorship will only work if it is carefully designed, and if well-thought out criteria are provided to guide preceptor selection and preparation. She stresses particular emphasis on promoting the principles of adult learning theory, clinical teaching strategies and methods of performance evaluation.

One difference to bear in mind in the British proposals for preceptorship is that of the support aspects of the relationship.

In the USA, the primary emphasis appears to be on improved role performance as an outcome of successful preceptoring: in UKCC 'speak' higher levels of competence seem to be viewed more as an extremely important byproduct of the support offered by the new system, as a logical *consequence* of support. This could have profound implications for the measurement of performance criteria in newly qualified, appointed or returning nurses to the workplace in Britain.

Could a situation arise for example where a nurse may be well supported via preceptorship (so that some of the criteria for successful preceptoring are met), but still fail in an assessment of his/her technical competence? How, therefore, can performance be best assessed? And is it fair to attribute any shortcomings to the preceptorship process alone? It may not be that the relationship has failed, but that other constraints within the working environment have prevailed.

When it comes to formally assessing the preceptee, what will be considered as the crucial benchmark of her abilities, the dexterity with which she manages technological innovation or her ability to counsel and comfort a patient? Who will draw the dividing line between affective aspects of learning and those that are cognitive?

In a situation where the nurse is technically highly competent but unable to build a rapport with patients, where on the continuum from novice to expert will this person be found? There appears to be very little in the North American literature which addresses clearly the vital issue of ethical decision-making in peer support. It seems to be assumed by all parties that the qualified nurse is inherently capable of managing such a complex interaction with her peers – a notion far from borne out in the British nursing literature, which is testimony to the abject failure of the system (and of those nurses working within it) to provide the necessary clinical and emotional support for colleagues within their working environment (Stoter, 1992).

Jameton (1984) states that the moral value of a nursing skill rests ultimately on patient good, while the ability of professionals to pursue a particular skill may depend on its challenge and interest. This is amply demonstrated in Britain in the glamour and high status afforded complex medically dominated specialisms (such as 'high tech' surgery and intensive care), and the predominantly lower status afforded to so-called 'basic nursing', for example, in the care of the long-stay elderly mentally ill person (see Chapman, 1987).

Jameton also observes that our cultural conceptions of competence tend to be oriented to visible activities with tangible products. Taking this a step further, the criteria for measuring effective preceptoring will need to identify clearly the perceived and somehow tangible improvement of both the preceptor and preceptee's technical competence, any resulting increase in the self-confidence and self-esteem of both parties, and a measurable positive impact on the quality of patient care. This is a complex issue which has not been adequately addressed in the nursing literature internationally – perhaps because some of what a nurse does is in a sense indefinable.

It is precisely because of these multiple factors in competence, and the obligation of professionals to seek both minimal and ever-higher levels of competence, that Jameton doubts whether adherence to the principle of competence can ever be attempted meaningfully. Does this mean therefore that we have no alternative as nurses but to stay with inappropriate and arbitrary judgements about our colleagues' performance?

Benner (1984) speaks of the intuitiveness of the expert nurse and suggests that only by breaking down and examining what an apparently expert nurse does will we bring about understanding of what 'expertness' is and how it can be acquired. She believes that the systematic study of proficient and expert performance should make it possible to describe expert nursing performance and the resultant patient outcomes, and that this knowledge can then be used further to develop the scope of practice of nurses who wish to be and are capable of excellence.

She accepts that not all nurses have the ability to become experts, but insists that descriptions of excellence are the key to new clinical possibilities:

'When experts can describe clinical situations where their interventions made a difference, some of the knowledge embedded in
practice becomes visible. And with visibility, enhancement and
recognition of expertise becomes possible'.

(Benner, 1984, p. 36)

The opportunity for preceptorship is therefore about providing inexperienced nurses with the opportunity to observe experienced clinical
staff, and to closely examine, with their help, what it is that makes them
effective both interpersonally and in terms of clinical expertness.

Confusion with mentorship

Several authors have discussed the emergent confusion regarding support roles in British nursing practice, notably Palmer (1987), Morle
(1990) and Armitage & Burnard (1991).

The introduction of the concept of mentorship to pre-registration
education in the mid-1980s (ENB Circular 1987/28) and the definition of
mentor as a 'wise reliable counsellor' and 'experienced trusted adviser'
sowed the seeds for considerable confusion among nurses, in that the
wider connotations of mentorship for personal growth appeared to
recede in the face of other more pragmatic considerations such as formal assessment of competence.

It has been argued that the element of formal assessment does not rest
easily with the nurturing, self-actualizing aspects of the mentor role, and
that existing interpretations of mentorship, at least in the English context, are actually more descriptive of 'preceptorship' than of 'mentorship'.

Morle (1989) points out that the Project 2000 qualified nurse may
experience 'reality shock' which is not dissimilar to that experienced by
nurses in the USA, and that it might be wise for nurses to heed the
potential problems of supernumerary status by acknowledging the
benefits of preceptorship in the prevention of wastage from nursing
during early clinical experiences. She also suggests a closer examination
of options for peer support, such as 'buddying', whereby students are
paired with a fellow, more experienced student within the school or
faculty to help them adjust to new expectations.

If preceptorship, plus 'buddying', plus personal tutor support systems
were offered, then nurses might have the degree of support required to
enable them to function properly (Morle, 1989, p. 69).

Fortunately, the UKCC clarified the situation when it published its
formal 'position paper' outlining the Council's requirements for pre-

ceptor support, with the declared expectation that they should be implemented by employers of all practitioners by 1 April 1993.

The emphasis in the guidance is very clearly on the support aspects of the role, and the recognition that adjustment to new responsibilities is a gradual process which can be eased by the help and guidance of an experienced practitioner. The contents of the position paper are reproduced here to give you the background to the Council's thinking and rationale.

UKCC guidance on preceptor support

United Kingdom Central Council
for Nursing, Midwifery and Health Visiting

**The Council's position concerning a period of
support and preceptorship for nurses, midwives and health visitors
entering or re-entering registered practice**

The Council's policy:
(1)   The Council considers that all newly registered nurses, midwives and health visitors should be provided with a period of support for approximately the first four months of practice as a registered nurse, midwife or health visitor, under the guidance of a preceptor, and this is described in paragraphs 3 to 11.

(2)   The Council also considers that those practitioners returning to practise by virtue of a registered qualification in nursing, midwifery or health visiting, after a break of five years or more, should also be provided with a period of support based on the principles described below. The requirements for such returning practitioners are set out in paragraphs 13 to 15.

Newly registered nurses, midwives and health visitors:

The purpose of a period of support:
(3)   Starting practice as a registered nurse, midwife and health visitor offers a considerable challenge to newly registered practitioners, whether entering registered practice for the first time or entering practice by virtue of a second registerable qualification. It represents a major transition from student to professional practitioner. This period is a formative one in

which knowledge, skills and attitudes acquired during the pre-registration programme of education are applied in practice. It is a transition period which can be stressful as well as challenging, as new demands are made upon individuals who are seeking to practise their skills and accept responsibility as registered practitioners. It is, therefore, a period where the registered practitioner, although professionally competent at the minimum level of safety, is in need of guidance and support from more experienced practitioners. Such support and guidance will help to ensure responsibilities are not placed too soon or inappropriately upon a newly registered and inexperienced practitioner. The care and protection of patients and clients will be enhanced by these measures designed to support and develop practitioners who are engaged in their care.

Accountability:
(4) Individual practitioners will have achieved specific competencies or learning outcomes as part of the Council's requirements for registration. The period of support is not to be considered as an extension of the formal programme of education leading to registration. It is a means of providing support during the early months of registered practice. Nurses, midwives and health visitors will be accountable for their practice from the point of registration regardless of any support system. Local management should, of course, balance the level of responsibility with the experience of the individual.

Primary practice:
(5) The period of support should be distinguished from primary practice. The PREPP report defines primary practice as being able to accept responsibility with confidence, in co-operation with other practitioners and disciplines as required, for the individual's or group's health care needs. Such care will be comprehensive, appropriate and, where possible, based on relevant research. The nature of primary practice and its relationship to specialist and advanced practice will be subject to further elaboration once the Council's requirements for the standard, kind and content of post-registration education are known.

Who needs support?:
(6) The period of support should be available to all newly registered nurses, midwives and health visitors entering practice for the first time and for practitioners entering a different field of practice by means of a second registerable qualification. This applies to all areas of practice, whether in the National Health Service or in private or independent practice.

The length of the support period:
(7) The Council considers that the average period of support necessary for newly registered practitioners should be four months. This will be subject to local agreement and based upon the previous experience, qualifications and personal abilities of the individual concerned. At the end of the support period, practitioners should be able to meet the criteria for primary practice (as described in paragraph 5 above) in the opinion of the practitioner and the preceptor. Where this position is not reached within the

agreed period time, the length of the support period should be reviewed and, ultimately, the employer may need to reconsider the scope and direction of the individual's role, to ensure that they practise within the limits of their ability.

Role of preceptors:

(8) Preceptors will be first level nurses, midwives or health visitors who have had at least twelve months (or equivalent) experience within the same or associated clinical field as the practitioner requiring support. They may be full or part-time practitioners and will have shown a willingness and aptitude for the role as described below and be eager to share their knowledge and skills with those entering that field of professional practice.

(9) The preceptor should be seen as a guide and supporter for the newly registered practitioner; a colleague who can act as a valuable source of help, both professionally and personally during the early and uncertain months of registered practice. The exact nature of the role and relationship between practitioner and preceptor will be dependent upon the nature and context of the care to be given, the location and the experience and confidence of the practitioners concerned. The preceptor will recognise that the newly registered practitioner is accountable for their own actions within the context and limitations of their own knowledge as set out in Clause 4 of the Council's Code of Professional Conduct. The Council recognises and appreciates that this role is already being carried out in an informal way by many existing registered practitioners and that many examples of excellent practice exist already.

Preparation of preceptors:

(10) Preceptors will require specific preparation for their role. It is recognised, however, that many experienced nurses, midwives and health visitors will already have acquired some, if not all, of the necessary skills. It is anticipated that any additional specific preparation would not exceed a period of two days and that this may be more appropriately divided into smaller periods to be completed over a longer period to allow flexibility of preparation to meet the needs of the individual and the service. The outcomes of the preparation will be that the preceptor will:

10.1 have sufficient knowledge of the practitioner's programme leading to registration to identify current learning needs;

10.2 help the practitioner to apply knowledge to practice;

10.3 understand how practitioners integrate into a new practice setting and assist with this process;

10.4 understand and assist with the problems in the transition from pre-registration student to registered and accountable practitioner and

10.5 set, with the practitioner, objectives for learning to assist with this transition.

Determining the preceptor:

(11) The Council anticipates that, in some areas, preceptors will be identified from the immediate team within which the newly registered nurse, mid-

wife or health visitor is practising. In other instances it may be more practical or desirable that the preceptor is chosen from another associated area of practice. The Council considers that the most suitable arrangements for effective preceptorship should be defined locally taking account of the context of practice and the needs of the newly registered practitioner.

The position of practitioners not able to gain employment following registration:

(12) The period of support would be required at the time the newly registered practitioner enters registered practice and assumes responsibility as a registered nurse, midwife or health visitor. The Council recognises that, for a variety of reasons, this will not always be immediately following qualification.

Practitioners returning to practise after a beak:

(13) Where a practitioner is re-entering registered practice by virtue of a nursing, midwifery or health visiting qualification after a break of five years or more, a period of support is also required. This should follow completion of a return to practise programme. These programmes will become a statutory requirement and further details will be issued by the Council in due course.

(14) The purpose of a return to practise programme is to enable the practitioner to re-enter registered practice, following appropriate preparation, with confidence and renewed ability. A period of support, once practice begins, will contribute to the confidence of the 'returner', enhancing their practice and improving their contribution to care and to the team.

(15) The length of the period of support will be dependent upon the needs of the individual practitioner and the role which they will undertake.

Conclusion:

The Council and the Government Health Departments consider that the provision of a period of support and preceptorship is necessary and is good practice and expect steps to be taken to ensure that such arrangements, where not already in place, are implemented by appropriate authorities and employers of all nurses, midwives and health visitors from 1 April 1993.

It is interesting to note that in paragraph 4 the Council emphasizes that the (average) four-month period of support is 'not to be considered as an extension of the formal programme of education leading to registration'. Instead, it stresses that it is a means of providing support during the early months of registered practice and a preparation for 'primary practice' which in turn is described as:

'being able to accept responsibility with confidence, in co-operation with other practitioners and disciplines as required, for the individual's or group's health care needs. Such care will be comprehensive, appropriate and, where possible, based on relevant research.'

(UKCC, 1993).

In other words, the Council expects preceptors to set a good example, and preceptees to follow it in accordance with the Code of Professional Conduct (UKCC, 1992). Having defined *primary practice* the Council can go on, with further work, to consider and provide guidance on what constitutes specialist and advanced practice.

Whilst the definition of primary practice could be accused of being rather woolly and difficult to measure in concrete terms, it at least gives us a baseline from which to develop individual competencies which taken together could paint a portrait of the kind of practitioner required in order to take nursing forward in terms of practice and professional accountability.

Similarly, we now have some idea of who is considered to be good preceptor material, i.e. first-level nurses with at least twelve months (or equivalent) experience within the same or associated clinical field as the practitioner requiring support.

There is some flexibility in interpreting how preceptorship can be managed at local levels, with the statement allowing the exact nature of the role and relationship between practitioner and preceptor to be determined by the nature and context of the care to be given, the location, and the experience and confidence of the practitioners concerned.

Most importantly, the Council has taken pains to point out that the newly registered practitioner is accountable for her own actions within the context and limitations of her own knowledge as set out in Clause 4 of the Council's Code of Professional Conduct. Presumably the UKCC could argue that the preceptor is already bound by the Code of Conduct and particularly the clause which requires practitioners to be mindful of their responsibilities to colleagues to ensure that they are not given too much or inappropriate responsibility.

Preceptor selection and preparation

Although no specific guidance is given on preceptor selection, potential preceptors can be drawn from full- and part-time practitioners provided they have 'shown a willingness and aptitude for the role' and are eager to 'share their knowledge and skills' with those entering that field of professional practice.

This is interesting and an aspect of the requirement which is usually met with scorn and derision from staff nurses who assume that, as in the case of Myrick's 'warm body syndrome', the scarcity of available staff who meet the 12 months' experience criteria is likely to severely restrict the number of first-level practitioners able to fulfil the preceptor role.

Notions of being pressured to undertake such a role are difficult to assuage, but they will need to be addressed urgently if we are to have a chance of implementing the recommendation in a civilized way. The Council is keen to 'recognize and appreciate' that the preceptor role is already being carried out in an informal way, and that many examples of excellent practice exist already.

In the case of preceptorship, however, at least one task is now made easier in the UK: that of measuring outcomes to the preceptor process. If we accept that preceptor support is primarily about improving the new nurses' confidence to perform, rather than performance itself, we can begin to judge the success of preceptorship by its impact on the emotional careers of practitioners and not simply on their 'hands on' skills. The US literature on preceptorship has a strong tendency to focus on psychomotor and cognitive aspects of role development, and thus misses out on what might be the most enlightening study of all – that of the effect of emotions on a practitioner's ability to come to terms with a new role and responsibilities.

Given that health care is, above all, a human service, it seems reasonable, if somewhat overdue, to be looking more closely at the affective domain of learning. In this way, we can begin to examine our responses to emotional stressors and perhaps determine new and more acceptable ways of dealing with those that pose us with the greatest problems.

Affective aspects of education could then be perceived as a legitimate subject for study, instead of being relegated to the lower ranking 'qualitative side' of educational theory. Because an approach is qualitative rather than quantitative it is sometimes accused of being too 'soft' or 'unscientific'.

Preceptor support is a golden opportunity for educational researchers and practitioners to explore what is meant when we say someone has an 'aptitude' for teaching or nursing, and to address the issue in a systematic as well as intuitive way. The criteria developed locally to determine who has an 'aptitude' for the preceptor role are a fascinating subject for study which would benefit from wider discussion and debate as to our values and beliefs about what being supportive means. The notion of distancing oneself from any emotional interaction with patients and clients as a form of self-protection could then be examined to see whether in fact it is actually successful in protecting us as professional carers, or whether in reality we may be causing ourselves unnecessary emotional stress by denying our involvement with fellow human beings.

It surely follows that if preceptorship can enable us to become more understanding and supportive of our colleagues, then similar values could be carried in to our day-to-day work, and help us to communicate more fully (and perhaps more honestly) with those people who place such faith and trust in us at times of crisis and transition in *their* lives.

We also need to be careful when selecting staff to be preceptors not to assume automatically that because someone appears capable they will necessarily want to undertake the additional responsibility. Nurse managers will need to be sympathetic to the fact that 12 months' experience is not really very long, and that individuals will have their own feelings and perceptions about how confident they may be to work closely with a new member of staff over the four months or so required of the preceptorship.

Careful discussion and explanation of the responsibilities will be necessary if the would-be preceptor is to give his/her informed consent to undertaking the role planned.

Again, the UKCC has tried to be fairly open in its recommendation that specific preparation for the role should not exceed two days, but that this 'may be more appropriately divided into smaller periods over a longer period to allow flexibility of preparation to meet the needs of the individual and the service'.

At best, this would seem ambitious; at worst, wholly inadequate. There is a danger, here, that with all the pressures currently confronting managers in practice the preceptor requirement will be paid only 'lip service', and that the skills of an effective preceptor will be largely assumed rather than acquired. In recognizing the need to formalize support the Council has made it clear that it is not only staff who are to benefit from the new requirement, but the consumer, too. It is vital, therefore, that whoever has overall or delegated responsibility for implementing the new policy – whether based in the clinical or academic setting – takes the preparation and on-going support of preceptors very seriously. To do otherwise would be to miss the point of the exercise altogether, and to perpetuate past experience by adding to the individual's workload and responsibilities without due regard for its pressures.

The existing literature on preceptorship shows clearly that nothing can be taken for granted when it comes to learning how to practice with confidence, and to attempt to take short-cuts in preparation is to take heavy risks in the policy being successful, not to mention the human costs in terms of wasted energies, disillusionment and unnecessary mistakes.

With proper planning and standardization of a core curriculum for preceptorship, it is possible to provide cost-effective preparation which, in turn, is likely to reap rewards in terms of greater job satisfaction and subsequent retention of staff in the clinical area. Whether or not it improves measurably, the latter would be a valuable area of empirical research.

The UKCC is, of course, aware of the cost constraints within the service and is attempting to be realistic in the face of all the other recommendations for post-registration education and practice contained in its 'PREPP' report (for more information please see UKCC, 1990 'Summary of Recommendations').

The preceptor requirement is only one of several equally important demands in respect of continuing nurse education in the UK, and, as such, it has to be implemented as inexpensively as possible if any other requirements are to stand a chance of obtaining the government funding necessary for their implementation nationally.

In determining preceptor preparation therefore we are going to have to provide the strongest argument possible if we are to harness the resources necessary to enable us to extend support not only to those identified by the UKCC, but to all staff undergoing role change who are equally deserving of such support. The strongest argument possible is evidence that preceptorship works, and that its rewards are tangible and visible in terms of better retention, higher morale, and an increased sense of purpose and mission in improving the quality of care provided to patients.

It isn't enough to say that we will attempt to do the best we can with whatever resources may be available locally, although we will have to begin by formulating soundly researched models of good practice which will encompass the outcomes of preparation outlined by the UKCC's guidelines. Perhaps it should be remembered that the outcomes suggested can only provide a framework for future practice, and that it is up to individuals to work cohesively to piece together the jigsaw that comprises personal and professional development.

Preceptorship is, after all, only a beginning stage to professional practice which is important because it sets the tone for future professional relationships.

While it is important to be pragmatic and realistic, therefore, we can still pursue the ideal by setting targets and looking further ahead to see where else an approach to learning can take us with respect to individual growth and professional growth as a whole.

Formal requirements for preceptor preparation

The UKCC states that:

> 'The outcome of the preparation will be that the preceptor will:

- Have sufficient knowledge of the practitioner's programme leading to registration to identify current learning needs;
- Help the practitioner to apply knowledge to practice;
- Understand how practitioners integrate into a new practice setting and assist with this process;
- Understand and assist with the problems in the transition from pre-registration student to registered and accountable practitioner;
- Set, with the practitioner, objectives for learning to assist with this transition'.

How we go about providing preparation in order to obtain these outcomes is left to professionals themselves to ascertain.

The most critical and potentially problematic issue may be that of adopting formal peer assessment, whereby the preceptor assesses and judges the preceptee's preparedness for primary practice – not to be confused here with primary nursing, which is an entirely different concept – on the basis of two days' training. This may cause some anxiety in the service and we will need to weigh up the pros and cons very carefully if we are not to discourage staff from taking up the preceptor role.

Problems of assessment

The thorny issue of who decides when a practitioner is ready to assume the responsibilities of primary practice is alluded to in paragraph 7 of the UKCC's position paper, which says that at the end of the support period, practitioners should be able to meet the criteria for primary practice in the opinion of the practitioner and the preceptor:

> 'Where this is not reached within the agreed period of time, the length of the support period should be reviewed and, ultimately, the employer may need to reconsider the scope and direction of the individual's role, to ensure that they practise within the limits of their ability'.

This could be interpreted as being perilously close to asking the preceptor to judge whether the preceptee is safe to practice or not; something which should have been determined prior to registration. The

UKCC's assertion that the period of support is not to be considered as an extension of the formal programme of education leading to registration is thus placed in jeopardy; as is the principle of support.

The concept of support (which is to be open, non-judgemental, and enabling) is in direct conflict with that of assessing a person's performance and recommending whether or not that person is now ready to assume the greater responsibilities of first level practice. Assessment is by its nature subjective and open to distortion. Ramsden (1992) has some salutary comments to make on making expectations clear to those being assessed (and presumably to the assessor!), and on encouraging student autonomy.

He advocates the use of clear and unambiguous language to reduce the debilitating anxiety that assessment can impose on learners:

> 'There need to be no apprehension of reducing a student's anxiety too much: if a learner desires to understand, that inner pressure will always provide enough tension ... good teaching helps students to become aware that educationally valid assessment is an opportunity to learn and to reveal the depth of one's knowledge'.

> (Ramsden, 1992, p. 197)

Consistent effort will therefore need to be made to ensure that preceptors have the skills, knowledge and interpersonal attributes required to make educationally valid assessments of their preceptees.

Assessors will also need to recognize, as Dawson (1022) says, that the attempted measurement of attitude in nursing education is an inherently dangerous occupation which should not rely on the outcomes of simplistic behavioural tools. Any such measurement is based on attitudes towards the *activity* being examined, and cannot be taken as a measurement of attitudes as a whole – a fact not always acknowledged and allowed for in practice-based assessment.

Developing a workable curriculum model for practice

Promoting change from within

For those employed as continuing educators in nursing it requires a certain singularity of purpose to find space for practice innovation in the midst of all-embracing change.

The introduction of the 'nursing process' to Britain in the late 1970s was a splendid example of how continuing educators can get it hideously wrong when attempting to change problems in practice by imposing solutions from *outside the context* in which changes were to be implemented.

The lesson for continuing educators from this debacle, was that change, to be successful, has to come from *within*. It must be a shared activity in which all the individuals involved take some responsibility for identifying needs and problems, for working out practical solutions to them together, while at the same time benefiting from the educational processes which can occur at the same time. An important prerequisite to this is a critical analysis of the concepts which are being offered to 'learners' in a given situation.

The term 'curriculum', for example, is defined in the Shorter Oxford English Dictionary as a 'course', i.e. a 'regular course of study as at a school' (SOED, p. 474).

Jarvis (1983, p. 211) says that it is a word rarely used in the education of adults, most adult educators preferring to use the term 'programme' to differentiate between the content of a particular subject area, and its use as a description of the whole programme of learning offered by an educational institution.

Gosby (1989, p. 65) provides a useful overview of 'curricula' when she sets down four 'generally accepted descriptions' or classifications of curricula as:

(1) The official curriculum: that reflecting the statutory requirements of education and training;
(2) The formal curriculum: the detailed syllabus, allocation programme and selection of teaching strategies determined by educationalists;
(3) The actual curriculum: the actual teaching and learning that takes place, which may not actually reflect either of the above;
(4) The hidden curriculum: described as the transmission of attitudes and values from teacher to student or from the institution where learning takes place.

The term 'model' in relation to curriculum is also an interesting subject for study. Tight (1985, p. 3) says that the creation and elaboration of models generally represents an attempt towards finding order.

A conceptual 'model' or framework can be defined as a way of looking at a subject or area in a clear unambiguous way that can be communicated to others' (Martin, 1987, p. 49), but the relationship *between* theories and models is also important, as Tight explains:

'Whereas theories endeavour to make clear the meanings of phenomena, models merely aim to represent them. Models may, of course, draw upon theories and, if successful, can be expected to provide the basis for further theory development'.

(Tight, 1985, p. 5)

A suggested curriculum model of preceptorship for clinical practice

We have had to make some imaginative leaps into the dark in the formulation of a model of preceptorship that stands a chance of being implemented in the current climate of change and severe financial constraints. The model offered is immediately acknowledged as untried and therefore purely theoretical at this stage, although continuing research into its effectiveness is currently taking place. (Morton-Cooper, 1992b').

What is vitally important is that we attempt to grasp, even at this stage in the concept's infancy in the UK, the extent to which preceptorship may influence not only the support offered to new practitioners but also the expansion and dissemination of the broader principles of adult-centred and self-directed learning in continuing education within the health service.

All aspects of the service stand to benefit from a more integrated workforce; nursing particularly needs to regain its focus on how both qualified and unqualified nursing staff can expect to develop simultaneously alongside one another in a demanding and complex learning environment.

With more nurses beginning to specialize in staff and professional development, it is essential that we maintain a strategic view of where the service is going in terms of its contribution to total patient care. Service delivery mechanisms will have to include:

- The direct provision of continuing education services;
- Effective planning and co-ordination of all those involved;
- Collaboration across the institutions concerned;
- Consultation with those who stand to be affected by the changes proposed;
- Support for those negotiating and facilitating change.

(Kelly, 1992, p. 43)

Preceptors and those who educate and manage them will need to take account of what has already been learned about adult approaches to teaching and learning, and about theoretical concepts which underpin practice in the area of staff development, cited by Kelly (1992, p. 29) as:

- Adult learning and education;
- Change theory;
- Human resource development theory;
- Nursing itself;
- Organization development;
- Systems development.

Preceptor activities and accountability

We do need to be realistic in what we ask of staff already burdened by multiple responsibilities. For this reason, while close collaboration and

(a)

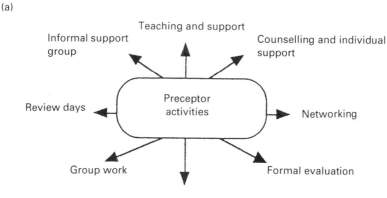

(b)

- Teaching and support in the clinical area at times to be agreed in the learning contract
- Group work as appropriate and planned with preceptees and fellow designated preceptors
- Review days within the institution and associated college department
- Informal support groups
- Counselling and individual support as prescribed within the preceptorship programme
- Formal evaluation via reflective learning diaries, critical incident techniques and practice based assessments
- Networking across the ward/area/unit and across institution and college
- Publication and dissemination of research and practice in preceptorship across the professions

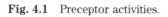

Fig. 4.1   Preceptor activities.

involvement of ward, unit, community, and senior nurse managers is envisaged in planning for implementation of the preceptor requirement, on-going responsibility for overseeing the system and preceptor functions should not be laid entirely at their door.

Instead, we propose that a unit preceptor be appointed as a programme co-ordinator of designated preceptors working within the clinical area (see Fig. 4.1). The designated preceptor may be of senior staff nurse level or above, but it needs to be borne in mind that many nurses find colleagues close to them in the hierarchy very approachable. Nurses who are newly appointed or newly returned to practice after a break in service like to make a good impression on their managers, and appreciate time to familiarize themselves with the logistics of the work area through a less senior member of staff before taking on any real responsibility (Morton-Cooper, 1988).

In a study of the ideal attributes of a ward teacher, Marson (1981) found that nurses were able to learn better when they felt they were accepted members of the ward team. However, 67% of the students interviewed by Marson reported feelings of reluctance to discuss problems of an emotional nature with the ward sister.

According to Lewis (1990), the role of the ward sister as 'professional gatekeeper' is such that 'for good or bad, the personal philosophy of the sister will set the tone of the ward and care within it' (p. 808). As such s/he has the power to bring about change or to maintain the status quo. The influence and contribution of the senior nurse is therefore critical for success (Ogier, 1989; Orton, 1981).

Given that in the early months after qualification or appointment the new nurse is likely to experience peaks and troughs of emotion as she gets to grips with her new responsibilities, it might be as well to have designated ward (or field-based) preceptors who are able to act as effective role models, but who do not overwhelm their preceptees by their vast experience and seniority (see Fig. 4.2).

The criteria for the selection of the *unit* preceptor on the other hand will need to be adapted to help those already working in a fairly senior role to assume responsibility for managing designated preceptors within their unit or area, and for negotiating time and resources with service and education managers for the on-going preparation and support of those preceptors.

The unit preceptor will have to acquire a sound understanding of staff development and adult learning, of counselling skills and the management of role conflict in the clinical area. Costs of initial preparation for the role and that of time to disseminate information with regard to the introduction of such a support system will need to be carefully assessed in consultation with colleagues who have direct

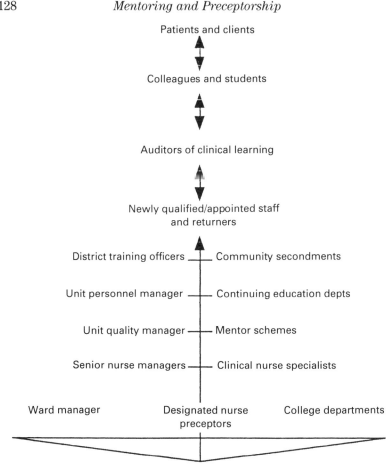

Patients and clients

Colleagues and students

Auditors of clinical learning

Newly qualified/appointed staff
and returners

District training officers ——— Community secondments

Unit personnel manager ——— Continuing education depts

Unit quality manager ——— Mentor schemes

Senior nurse managers ——— Clinical nurse specialists

Ward manager   Designated nurse   College departments
                          preceptors

Unit preceptor

Fig. 4.2 A curriculum model of preceptorship: unit preceptorship account-ability.

responsibility for teaching and research in both pre- and post-registra-tion education.

They will have a good idea of the amount of time it takes to prepare individuals for practice as clinical assessors, but they will also have to respect the nurse manager's need to account for every minute of every hour of seconded time, and every pound of continuing education money spent.

The content of the suggested preparatory workshops is based on findings in the literature, and on experience of working with practi-tioners who are often studying for other advanced qualifications in addition to their everyday clinical work (see Fig. 4.3).

Teaching and learning	Skills and actions

Adult teaching and learning strategies
The constructive use of learning
Contracts and learning needs
    assessment
Teaching and assessing in the clinical
    learning environment
Evaluation and monitoring of the
    learning process/environment
	Leadership and effective role modelling
	Communication and support skills
	Concepts and skills of self and peer
	    assessment/evaluation of
	    performance

Management	**Professional development**

Self and time
Concepts and practice of organizational
    management and change
Professional/bureaucratic conflict
Management of teaching and assessing
    in the clinical learning environment
	Introduction to socialization processes
	Principles of anticipatory socialization
	Ethical concepts and the precepting
	    relationship
	Concepts of staff and professional
	    development
	Accountability and preceptor function

Fig. 4.3 Suggested workshop format.

Learning needs, assessment and preceptor preparation

Haberlin (1983) suggests two ways of preparing preceptors, either on an individual basis or in a group situation. The advantage of the latter is the formation of an immediate peer group and a sharing of issues and anxieties concerning the preceptorship. It also gives the programme co-ordinator or supervisor an opportunity to observe the 'social style and interactive patterns' of individual preceptors as they relate to other members of the group (Haberlin, 1983, p. 49).

Individualized preparation, whilst an expensive and time-consuming option, might give greater flexibility and it gives the potential preceptor practice at establishing rapport with an individual where the relationship will be similar to that of the preceptor relationship itself.

To do this effectively, however, probably requires more resources than most departments have available. It needn't be ruled out, however, and could be fitted in to a standardized preceptor programme, perhaps as part of the planning and evaluation process.

The business of assessing learning needs can be a complex process requiring skill and sound techniques. There is the ever-present temptation in the clinical environment either to presume needs on the basis of previous anecdotal experience, or to impose learning (by way of 'content' and input) on the basis of organizational demands. This needs to be approached with caution, however, or there is the danger that money and time can be invested inappropriately with ineffectual results.

Puetz (1992) describes three key elements in the learning needs assessment which make up a framework for the process:

- Investigation
- Validation
- Communication

In the context of the workplace, *investigation* is the search for learning needs 'that must be met in order for nursing staff to perform to an expected and defined standard, and to meet the organization's missions and goals' (Puetz, 1992, p. 98).

Puetz puts forward Knowles' definition of the staff development role in helping adults discover and become interested in meeting their real needs, rather than just their interests (Knowles, 1980). The tension in staff development in differentiating between the two, and finding the acceptable dividing line between personal and professional development is certainly a challenge for those working in staff development, particularly when the individual holds the view that the two are not mutually exclusive.

Validation is the second stage of the learning needs assessment process and is required to identify the exact nature of the learning needs, and to ascertain whether they are in fact learning needs or a symptom of problems elsewhere in the organization, such as poor communication, misunderstanding, unrealistic expectations or lack of adequate supervision. If the need can be attributed to any of the above then it is not helped solely by providing input, but rather by pinpointing the difficulties and bringing them to the attention of people who can rectify the situation.

Validation uses techniques such as questionnaires, interviews, group discussion and nominal group technique, individual appraisals and other more sophisticated techniques described in detail in two excellent books edited by Kelly (1992) and Abbruzzese (1992), respectively. (Both texts give a comprehensive overview of staff development strategies in relation to nursing, and are a rich resource for the continuing educator.)

Validation is therefore about targeting continuing education resources to where they are most needed, and about making decisions about provision on the basis of valid assessments. The technique of 'triangulation' – whereby a number of techniques are employed to derive the same information – is a helpful tool to guide the content and process of a curriculum, and preceptorship programmes could benefit from time devoted to it at an early stage.

The final stage of assessment is *communication*. Puetz believes that this is the time for communicating the outcome of a needs assessment so that staff are clear about what is happening and are in a good position to know about proposed staff development activities well in advance. Communication strategies by way of newsletters, bulletin boards, reports and in-service meetings which demonstrate the link between practice and continuing education can help to raise awareness among staff and 'sensitize them to learning needs' in the process (Puetz, 1992, p. 100).

The ability to maintain a strategic view is one of the characteristics of a 'health organization' (Beckhard, cited in Broome, 1990), and helps motivate staff towards the development of a good climate for learning, typified by mutual respect and support, openness and authenticity, support and collaboration (Orton, 1979, cited in Marson *et al.*, 1981).

When planning to meet the learning needs of preceptors and their preceptees it is important not to lose sight of the broader strategic view, as it can help us to avoid blind alleys and investing too much energy on relatively unimportant matters while the real work goes untouched.

This is particularly true now that the four national boards have proposed their own routes to advanced practice, and that increasing numbers of nurses are undertaking degree level work both in nursing and in health service and resource management. Care needs to be taken to see that practitioners are not overloaded in the quest for higher standards of practice, or the ultimate consequences may be a perception of personal failure which, in turn, equates with professional failure and the very 'reality shock' we are attempting to reduce.

Continuing support through regular review days and appropriate documentation of learning between preceptors and their preceptees is, of course, important, and can be facilitated by negotiated learning plans, contracts and agreements, and by formal and informal support groups meeting regularly at an appropriate time and venue.

Increasing use is being made of individualized learning contracts, reflective diaries and critical incident techniques to assess the effects of newly acquired learning (and the learning process) on the patient care provided (e.g. Dudley Road Management Development Programme, 1992).

Evaluation of the outcome of preceptorship have yet to be measured and widely documented in British nursing. The evaluation and continued debate as to the success of any support system is an exciting and enlightening part of ensuring quality in support provision. The search for reliable tools to measure its effects therefore requires lengthy discussion with quality assurance staff and with preceptees to see where it can be utilized best and fitted in with other local and national support networks, especially with regard to other support roles. Audit of the clinical learning environment is one obvious area for the exploration of learning support systems (see Reed & Price, 1991).

An example of a learning needs analysis exercise

A study to assess the needs of preceptors both before and after the preceptor experience was carried out in a 404 bedded urban teaching hospital in Boston, Massachusetts, USA. It asked 71 acute- and critical-care nurses to complete a 22-item questionnaire (rated on a five-point Likert scale) with descriptors ranging from (1) strong need, to (5) no need.

The questionnaire asked participants to respond to the statement 'to be a more effective preceptor I need more information/exposure to....' by rating 15 listed variables. Subjects were also asked to rate the same variables by responding to the statement 'I believe that *all* preceptors need information/exposure to....'

Half the questionnaire therefore addressed the individual preceptor's needs, while the other half measured the change in the preceptor's opinion of what content and preparation was considered to be essential for all preceptors to have. The researchers point out that participants represented various levels of educational preparation and years of nursing practice.

The study found that there were differences in perceived needs on two of the 15 items, namely, that more guidance on evaluating novice performance was required, together with the perceived need for more clinical experience in order to function well as a preceptor:

> 'We recognized that evaluating novice performance was critical to the preceptor role and a key to successful novice orientation. Most preceptors have little or no experience of teaching their nursing colleagues. Therefore, the preceptor workshop content places a strong emphasis on adult teaching learning principles with a particular focus on evaluating novice performance'

> (Westra & Graziano, 1992, p. 213)

The authors concluded that preceptor preparation should include a comprehensive educational effort which placed emphasis on the above, and which helped preceptors to assess an individual's learning needs, identify learning styles and 'readiness' and motivation to learn, and taught them how to provide feedback to the learner by suggesting teaching strategies appropriate for the clinical area.

In a further study which looked at the themes considered important to the development of the preceptor relationship Hsieh & Knowles (1990) found that *trust* came highest on the list, followed by *clearly defined expectations, support systems, honest communication, mutual respect and acceptance, encouragement, and mutual sharing of self and experience*, in short, what Palmer would describe as an 'enabler' (Palmer, 1993).

Hsieh & Knowles also examined the variables affecting the relationship, which included:

● Compatibility of personalities;
● Familiarity with the nursing programme;
● Budget cutbacks;
● Registered nurse 'burnout' or job dissatisfaction;
● Lack of assertion in the preceptor or preceptee;
● Conflicting values;
● Personal problems;
● Awareness, co-operation and support of peers;
● The self-confidence of preceptor and preceptee;
● The flexibility and creativity of the preceptor and preceptee.

The five likely variables which are not included in the list above but which would merit further study in the British context are:

● Nature of the clinical environment/workplace;
● Educational background of both parties;
● Nature of the job the new employee is undertaking;
● Attitude and support of clinical line managers;
● Extent and kind of preparation both individuals receive in anticipation of the preceptorship.

The content of any proposed learning and its accessibility (i.e. learning style, facilities, access to libraries etc) would presumably also have an impact. The absence of such factors from Hsieh's study are probably largely due to the fact that the preceptees in this case are students approaching qualification and are therefore supported by college, rather than in the UK where they are qualified and may or may not be receiving support from educationalists.

This is an important point to remember when looking at the methodologies and results of North American studies on precepting and their potential applications in the UK setting.

Theoretical underpinnings of the curriculum

The model offered here is based on the premise put forward by Kolb that 'learning is *the* major process of human adaptation' (Kolb, 1993, p. 149). Such experiential learning takes place in all human settings, across all 'life-stages', and, according to Kolb, encompasses other, more limited adaptive concepts, such as creativity, problem-solving, decision-making, and attitude change. All of these could be said to be helpful to the individual in learning to live with change and to make a positive adaptation to their social and physical environment (Fig. 4.4)

It is based on Rogers' view that the goal of education, if we are to survive, is the facilitation of change and learning; a humanistic, person-

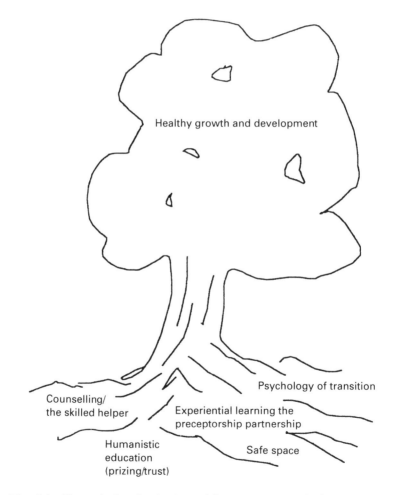

Fig. 4.4   Theoretical underpinnings of the preceptor curriculum.

centred form of education which concentrates on process and the ability to learn how to learn, rather than on prescriptive content determined by people working outside the context in which learning is intended to take place. As Rogers says, 'realness is the facilitator of learning' (Rogers, 1933, p. 231). In our view it is important not to be afraid of realness, and worth taking the risk of trying to identify shared values with colleagues if we are to try and make adaptation to new roles fluid, less stressful and above all rewarding.

Role theory and the dynamics of role conflict undoubtedly play a part in describing what happens to individuals when they perceive pressures to conform and respond to given situations. Gross *et al.* (1958), for example, describe role conflict as 'any situation in which the incumbent of a focal position perceives that he is confronted with incompatible expectations' (p. 248). Expectations can be considered both legitimate (and thought of as a rightful obligation), or illegitimate (considered unreasonable by the individual in the circumstances which prevail).

The need to examine and find strategies for dealing with role and value conflict is an integral part of providing support to staff in the workplace, as conflict can take several forms (see Hardy & Conway, 1988).

Theories of transition and change can also inform practice, so that people are prepared for change, and can begin to accept change as a vital ingredient in work and personal life (Broome, 1990; Wright, 1986).

The psychology of transition

This is a relative newcomer to the behavioural sciences and a fascinating subject for study when considering curriculum planning. Oatley (1990) has studied role transitions in relation to the emotional structures of everyday life, and has argued that emotions are in fact signals that accompany transitions between one kind of action and another. They function as alarm bells, and mark a potential transition between plans. When there is a transition between roles an emotion often occurs, either prompting transition or resulting from it. (See Oatley, 1990, p. 75 for further exploration of this hypothesis.)

The ability to manage such emotions and effect such transitions positively is the affective part of the learning process.

Nicholson (1990) has developed a taxonomy or classification of role transitions based on a cycle similar to Kolb's experiential learning theory. He describes it as a general framework which allows for the range of learners' experience, and one which can be used as a useful building-block for managing transitions.

The Nicholson transition cycle takes us from the preparation phase to the encounter, to adjustment and then to stabilization, on the basis that we will then be in a position to move forward to a new transition. The Nicholson model is particularly helpful in preceptorship implementation because of its cyclical strategies for effecting positive transitions. It requires thoughtful preparation and study before implementation, but nevertheless provides a valuable framework within which staff can learn to manage the stressful aspects of change effectively, while at the same time reducing the risk of dependency within the precepting relationship (see Nicholson, 1990, in Fisher & Cooper, 1990, pp. 83–108).

The concept of 'safe space'

Another concept which can be explored in relation to theories about human behaviour is that of Fry's 'safe space' (Fry, 1987). Anthony Fry is a consultant psychiatrist who believes that although our civilization and culture may change, our basic environmental requirements don't. Because the technological environment we have created for ourselves in order to provide for our energy needs, food and social structure has failed to keep us safe, we begin to feel threatened, the threat begins to permeate our consciousness and we begin to feel 'unsafe':

> 'In a polluted world, many natural cycles begin to fail. Cities and homes become evermore vulnerable and families and communities lose their stability. The hidden menace of Chernobyl lies in the soil waiting to be absorbed by the vegetables and meat that we shall eat this year and next year and for many, many years to come. The crime rates carry on rising, more and more children become victims of divorce, broken homes and abuse. Rates of mental illness, drug addiction and alcoholism go on rising. A common theme emerges – the world is becoming unsuitable for human consumption – the world is becoming unsafe'
>
> (Fry, 1987, p. 1)

Fry takes an ecological approach to the study of man's interaction with the environment, and suggests that the space in which we are, or which we create (whether it is material or personal), will profoundly affect not only the way we feel and function, but also our physical and mental health.

We therefore have to develop networks of social support which can sustain us in the face of perceived threat. Fry bases his strategy for support on four things, namely, *affection* (physical and emotional closeness), *affirmation* (the need to value ourselves and one another), *assessment* (preparedness to look for a second opinion, turning to friends, family and colleagues), and *aid* (providing and taking 'real' support).

This brings us back to the realness and genuineness suggested by Rogers earlier (Rogers, 1993). The atmosphere of colleagueship and 'kinship' we promote by preceptoring is therefore essentially about providing 'safe space', and generating a sense of self-worth which lessens any perceived sense of threat, and helps us to adjust to new or disorienting experiences.

Feeling safe can, paradoxically, give us the courage to take risks with our learning, and encourage us to think critically about our situation and our power to change things. Critical insight and a willingness to explore alternative ways of thinking and acting are part of becoming an analytical and critical thinker, and therefore an agent of change and an innovator (Brookfield, 1987).

Finally, the essence of the preceptor as the 'skilled helper' in assisting the preceptee to recognize and meet the professional demands made on her is worthwhile exploring, and one good reason for bringing the work of psychologist Gerard Egan into the preceptor curriculum.

Egan (1990) defines learning as taking place when options are increased: if collaboration between helpers and clients is successful, clients are likely to learn in a variety of ways, principally because they have more 'degrees of freedom' in their lives (Egan, 1990, p. 6).

All of these theories can inform the ethos and philosophy of the intended preceptor programme, and can help us to be creative in improving the quality of learning offered to beginning practitioners. It is necessary to be critical about adult educational theory, however, as the discipline is still relatively young and immature, and occasionally prone to hazy concepts and ill-disciplined analysis (see Davenport, 1993).

Like all theories, they are in some ways only as good as we feel them to be personally, and so that 'works' for one person may not relate to another very well. The best we can hope to expect from formal support roles in clinical practice is the encouragement of new learning within the confines of any 'safe space' which we may ultimately be successful in creating. Like any model, the one proposed is only one of many future interpretations.

Introducing preceptorship to clinical practice: a clinical resource file

This, the last part of the chapter, is intended to provide a clinical resource file which will help staff in clinical practice prepare themselves for the preceptor role, and educators provide the background reading necessary to formulate a workable curriculum model relevant to the work situation and clinical area.

In our experience, preceptorship models can be usefully linked to formal staff appraisal systems, and are easiest to implement when planned and delivered close to the clinical setting, i.e. within a nursing support team or staff development structure.

This is only one approach, however, and with the publication and dissemination of other models already functioning and developing elsewhere, the concept and its implications will no doubt continue to be explored and refined as appropriate to the setting.

Preparatory and background reading

The following suggestions are divided roughly into the topics or issues suggested for inclusion in the preceptor curriculum, and should be helpful for their use in 'ancestry' literature searching, i.e. the further reading and references given at the end of each article or chapter can be used to extend knowledge, and to provide suggestions as to how education and practice can be brought closer together.

Budgeting, costing and planning

Ham, C. (1991) *The New National Health Service: Organization and Management.* Radcliffe Medical Press, Oxford.

Healthcare Financial Management Association (1992) *Introductory Guide to NHS Finance.* HFMA/CIPFA, London.

Jones, T. & Prowle, M. (1987) *Health Service Finance: An Introduction.* The Certified Accountants Educational Trust, London.

Taylor, N. (1992) *Budgeting Skills: a Guide for Nurse Managers.* Quay Publishing Ltd, Lancaster.

Communication skills

Edwards, B.J. & Brilhart, J.K. (1981) *Communication in Nursing Practice.* CV Mosby Co, St Louis.

Janner, G. (1988) *Janner on Communications.* Century Hutchinson Business Books, London.

Macleod Nichol, N. & Walker, S. (eds) 1991) *Basic Management for Staff Nurses – A Companion to Practice.* Chapman and Hall, London. (See Chapter 2 'Communication'.)

Porritt, L. (1990) *Interaction Strategies – An Introduction for Health Professionals.* Churchill Livingstone, Edinburgh.

Vaughan, B. & Pillmoor, M. (eds) (1989) *Managing Nursing Work.* Scutari Press, London. (See Chapter 5 'Communication Networks'.)

Personal management skills

Allan, J. (1989) *How to Develop Your Personal Management Skills.* Kogan Page, London.
Bond, M. (1986) *Stress and Self-Awareness: A Guide for Nurses.* Heinemann Nursing, London.

Philosophical theories of education

Ozman, H. & Craver, S. (1990) *Philosophical Foundations of Education,* (4th edition). Merrill Publishing Company, Columbus, Ohio.
Russell, B. (1926) *On Education.* Unwin Hyman Ltd, London.
Trigg, R. (1988) *Ideas of Human Nature – an Historical Introduction.* Basil Blackwell, Oxford.

Adult education

Boud, D. (1981) *Developing Student Autonomy in Learning.* Kogan Page, London.
Brookfield, S. (1986) *Understanding and Facilitating Adult Learning.* The Open University, Milton Keynes.
Brookfield, S. (1987) *Developing Critical Thinkers: Challenging Adults to Explore Alternative Ways of Thinking and Acting.* Open University, Milton Keynes.
Cross, K.P. (1981 *Adults as Learners.* Jossey Bass, San Francisco
Jarvis, P. (1983) *Adult and Continuing Education – Theory and Practice.* Croom Helm, Beckenham.
Jarvis, P. (ed) (1987) *Twentieth Century Thinkers in Adult Education.* Routledge, London.
Marton, F., Hounsell, D. & Entwhistle, N. (eds) (1984) *The Experience of Learning.* Scottish Academic Press, Edinburgh.
Mezirow, J. (1990) *Fostering Critical Reflection in Adulthood: A Guide to Transformative and Emancipatory Learning.* Jossey Bass, San Francisco.
Rogers, A. (1986) *Teaching Adults.* The Open University, Milton Keynes.
Tight, M. (1985) *Adult Learning and Education.* Croom Helm, Beckenham.
Thorpe, M., Edwards, R. & Hanson, A. (eds) (1993) *Culture and Processes of Adult Learning.* Routledge/The Open University, London.
Walklin, L. (1990) *Teaching and Learning in Further and Adult Education.* Stanley Thornes Publishers, Cheltenham.
Westwood, S. & Thomas, J.E. (1991) *The Politics of Adult Education.* The National Institute of Adult, Continuing Education.

Professional education

Bines, H. & Watson, D. (eds) (1992) *Developing Professional Education.* The Open University, Milton Keynes.

Cervero, R.M. (1988) *Effective Continuing Education for Professionals.* Jossey Bass, San Francisco.

Houle, C.O. (1980) *Continuing Learning in the Professions.* Jossey Bass, San Francisco.

Jarvis, P. (1983) *Professional Education.* Croom Helm, Beckenham.

Goodlad, S. (ed) (1984) *Education for the Professions – Quis Custodiet.* SRHE and NFER Nelson, Guildford.

Clinical education

Benner, P. (1984) *From Novice to Expert: Excellence and Power in Clinical Nursing Practice.* Addison Wesley & Co., San Francisco.

Hinchliff, S. (ed) (1992) *The Practitioner as Teacher.* Scutari Press, London.

Kenworthy, N. & Nicklin, P. (1989) *Teaching and Assessing in Nursing Practice: An Experiential Approach.* Scutari Press, London.

Martin, L. (1989) *Clinical Education in Perspective.* Scutari Press, London.

McMahon, R. (ed) (1992) *Nursing at Night – A Professional Approach.* (See p. 149 'The Education of Nurses at Night'. Scutari Press, London.

Ogier, M.E. (1989) *Working and Learning – The Learning Environment in Clinical Nursing.* Scutari Press, London.

Perry, A. & Jolley, M. (eds) (1991) *Nursing – A Knowledge Base for Practice.* Edward Arnold, London.

Smith, P. *The Emotional Labour of Nursing – its Impact on Interpersonal Relations, Management and the Educational Environment in Nursing.* Macmillan, Basingstoke.

Preceptorships and nursing staff development

Abbruzzese, R.S. (ed) (1992) *Nursing Staff Development – Strategies for Success.* Mosby Yearbook, St Louis.

Armstrong, M. (1988) *A Handbook of Human Resource Management.* Kogan Page, London.

Dodwell, M. & Lathlean, J. (1989) *Management and Professional Development for Nurses.* Harper & Row, London.

Kelly, K.J. (ed) (1992) *Nursing Staff Development – Current Competence, Future Focus.* JB. Lippincott & Co., Philadelphia.

Leddy, S. & Pepper, J.M. (1989) *Conceptual Bases of Professional Nursing.* (2nd edition). J.B. Lippincott & Co, Philadelphia.

Marquis, B.L. & Huston, C.J. (1992) *Leadership Roles and Management Functions in Nursing: Theory and Applications.* J.B. Lippincott & Co, Philadelphia.

Morrow, K.L. (1984) *Preceptorships in Nursing Staff Development.* Aspen Systems Corporation, Rockville, Maryland.

Stuart-Siddall, S. & Haberlin, J.M. (1983) *Preceptorships in Nursing Education.* Aspen Systems Corporation, Rockville, Maryland.

Role theory and role analysis

Gross, N., Mason, W.S. & McEachern, A.W. (1958) *Explorations in Role Analysis*. John Wiley & Sons, New York.

Hardy, M. & Conway, M. (1988) *Role Theory – Perspectives for Health Professionals* (2nd edition). Appleton and Lange, California.

Psychology

Fisher, S. & Cooper, C.L. (eds) (1990). *On the Move: the Psychology of Change and Transition.* John Wiley & Sons, Chichester.

Tennant, M. (1988) *Psychology and Adult Learning.* Kogan Page, London.

Profiling and career planning

Brown, R.A. (1992) *Portfolio Development and Profiling for Nurses.* Quay Publishing Ltd, Lancaster.

Cormack, D.F.S. (ed) (1990) *Developing Your Career in Nursing.* Chapman and Hall, London.

Counselling and support skills

Burnard, P. (1989) *Counselling Skills for Health Professionals.* Chapman and Hall, London.

Egan, G. (1990) *The Skilled Helper – A Systematic Approach to Effective Helping.* Brooks/Cole Publishing Company, Pacific Grove, California.

Contract learning/assignments

Mazhhindu, G.N. (1990) Contract learning reconsidered: a critical examination of implications for application in nurse education. *Journal of Advanced Nursing*, **15**, pp. 101–109.

Neary, M. (1992) Contract assignments. *Senior Nurse*, **12** (4), pp. 14–17.

Assessment

Dunn, B. (1991) A caring curriculum. *Senior Nurse*, **11** (6), pp. 12–15.

Howard, D. (1991) Student profiles through action research. *Senior Nurse*, **11** (3), pp. 17–20.

Critical incident analysis

Dunn, W.R. & Hamilton, D.D. (1986) The critical incident technique – a brief guide. *Medical Teacher*, **8** (3), pp. 207–215.

Smith, A. & Russell, J. (1991) Using critical learning incidents in nurse education. *Nurse Education Today*, (11), pp. 284–91.

References

Abbruzzese, R.S. (1992) *Nursing Staff Development – Strategies for Success.* C.V. Mosby Co., New York.

Armitage, P. & Burnard, P. (1991) Mentors or preceptors? Narrowing the theory–practice gap. *Nurse Education Today,* **11**, 225–9.

Backenstose, P. (1983) in Stuart-Siddall, S., Haberlin, J.M. (eds) *Preceptorships in Nursing Education.* Aspen Systems Corporation, Rockville, Maryland, USA.

Benner, P. & Benner, R.V. (1979) *The New Nurses' Work Entry – A Troubled Sponsorship.* Tiresias Press, New York.

Benner, P. (1984) *From Novice to Expert: Excellence and Power in Clinical Nursing Practice.* Addison Wesley, California.

Brookfield, S.D. (1987) *Developing Critical Thinkers – Challenging Adults to Explore Alternative Ways of Thinking and Acting.* The Open University, Milton Keynes.

Broome, A.K. (1990) *Managing Change.* Macmillan, Basingstoke.

Chapman, C. (1987) *Sociology for Nurses.* Baillière-Tindall, London.

Chickerella, B.G. & Lutz, W.J. (1981) Professional nurturance: preceptorships for undergraduate nursing students. *American Journal of Nursing,* **1**, 107–109.

Clayton, G.M., Broome, M.E. & Ellis, L.A. (1989) Relationship between a preceptorship experience and role socialization of graduate nurses. *Journal of Nursing Education,* **28**, 2, 72–5.

Cruz, S. & Riley, G. (1984) Dual preceptorship. *Focus on Critical Care,* **11**, 5, 51–5.

Davenport, J. (1993) Is there any way out of the andragogy morass? in Thorpe, M., Edwards, R. & Hanson, A. (eds) *Culture and Processes of Adult Learning.* Routledge/The Open University, Milton Keynes.

Dawson, K.P. (1992) Attitude and assessment in nurse education. *Journal of Advanced Nursing,* **17**, 473–9.

Dobbie, B.J. & Karlinsky, N. (1982) A self-directed clinical practicum. *Journal of Nursing Education,* **21**, 9, 39–41.

Douville, M. (1983) in Stuart Siddall, S. & Haberlin, J.M. (eds) *Preceptorship in Nursing Education.* Aspen Systems Corporation, Rockville, Maryland, USA.

Dudley Road Hospital (1992) *Proposals for the Development of Ward Managers: Strategy for Nursing Document.* Acute unit, Dudley Road Hospital, Birmingham.

Egan, G. (1990) *The Skilled Helper: A Systematic Approach to Effective Helping,* (4th ed). Brooks Cole Publishing, California.

ENB, (1987) Circular 1987/28/MAT, *Institutional and Course Approval/Reapproval Process, Information Required, Criteria and Guidelines,* English National Board, London.

Fry, A. (1987) *Safe Space.* Dent, London.

Gosby, J. (1989) The development of nursing curricula in Bradshaw, P.L. *Teaching and Assessing in Clinical Nursing Practice.* Prentice-Hall, New York.

Gross, N., Mason, W.S. & McEachern, A.W. (1958) *Explorations in Role Analysis*. John Wiley & Sons, New York.

Haberlin, J.M. (1983) in Stuart-Siddall, S. & Haberlin, J.M. (eds) *Preceptorships in Nursing Education*. Aspen Systems Corporation, Rockville, Maryland, USA.

Hardy, M.E. & Conway, M.E. (1988) *Role Theory – Perspectives for Health Professionals* (2nd edition). Appleton and Lange, Norwalk, Connecticut/San Mateo, California.

Hitchings, K.S. (1989) Preceptors promote competence and retention: strategies to achieve success. *The Journal of Continuing Education in Nursing*, **20**, 6, 255–60.

Hsieh, N.L. & Knowles, W.D. (1990) Instructor facilitation of the preceptorship relationship in nursing education. *Journal of Nursing Education*, **6**, 262–8.

Huber, M.L. (1981) *The Effect of Preceptorship and Internship Orientation Programs on Graduate Nurse Performance*. Unpublished PhD thesis, Wayne State University, Michigan, USA.

Jairath, N., Costello, J., Wallace, P. & Rudy, L. (1991) The effect of preceptorship upon diploma program nursing students' transition to the professional nursing role. *Journal of Nursing Education*, **6**, 251–5.

Jameton, A. (1984) Competence: nurses have an obligation to be competent. *Nursing Practice: The Ethical Issues*, pp. 80–88. Prentice Hall, New Jersey, USA.

Jarvis, P. (1983) *Professional Education*. Croom Helm, London.

Kelly, K.J. (ed) (1992) *Nursing Staff Development: Current Competence and Future Focus*. JB Lippincott & Co., Philadelphia.

Knowles, M.S. (1980) *The Modern Practice of Adult Education: From Pedagogy to Andragogy* (2nd edition). Cambridge Books, New York.

Kolb, D.A. (1993) The process of experiential learning, in Thorpe, M , Edwards, R. & Hanson, A. (eds), *Culture and Processes of Adult Learning*. Routledge/ The Open University, London.

Kramer, M. (1974) Postgraduation nurse socialization: an emergent theory in *Reality Shock: Why Nurses Leave Nursing*, C.V. Mosby & Co., St. Louis.

Laschinger, H.K.S. & MacMaster, E. (1992) Effect of pregraduate preceptorship experience on development of adaptive competencies of baccalaureate nursing students, *Journal of Nursing Education*, **31**, 6, 258–64.

Lewis, K.E. (1986) What it takes to be a preceptor. *L'Infirmière Canadienne*, **7**, 18–19.

Lewis, T. (1990) The hospital ward sister: professional gatekeeper. *Journal of Advanced Nursing*, **15**, 808–18.

Limon, S., Bargagliotti, A. & Spencer, J.B. (1982) Providing preceptors for nursing students: what questions should you ask? *Journal of Nursing Administration*, **6**, 16–19.

Magill, M.K., France, R.D. & Munning, K.A. (1986) Educational Relationships. *Medical Teacher*, **8**, 2, 149–53.

Marson, S.N. (1981) *Ward Teaching Skills – An Investigation into the Beha-*

vioural Characteristics of Effective Ward Teachers. Unpublished MPhil thesis, Sheffield City Polytechnic.

Martin, P. (1987) *Psychiatric Nursing – A Therapeutic Approach.* Macmillan, Basingstoke.

Morle, K.M.F. (1990) Mentorship – is it a case of the emperor's new clothes or a rose by any other name? *Nurse Education Today,* **10**, 66–9.

Morton-Cooper, A. (1988) *The Needs of Nurse Returners: A Consumer Study.* Internal report, Macmillan, Basingstoke.

Morton-Cooper, A. (1992a) *An Evaluation of Preceptorship as an Appropriate Conceptual Model for British Continuing Nurse Education.* MEd dissertation, University of Warwick.

Morton-Cooper, A. (1992b) *The Effects of a Preceptorship Model of Learning Suppport on the Transition from Student to Accountable Practitioner.* MPhil/PhD research study. Continuing Education Research Centre, University of Warwick.

Morton-Cooper, A. (1993) *Expectations of the Preceptor Relationship.* West Midlands Regional Health Authority Conference paper. National Exhibition Centre, Birmingham.

Myrick, F. (1988) Preceptorship – is it the answer to the problems in clinical teaching? *Journal of Nursing Education,* **27**, 3, 136–8.

Nicholson, N. (1990) The transition cycle: causes, outcomes, processes and forms in Fisher, S. & Cooper, C.L. (eds) *On the Move: the Psychology of Change and Transition.* John Wiley & Sons, Chichester.

Oatley, K. (1990) Role transitions and the emotional structure of everyday life in Fisher, S. & Cooper, C.L. (eds) *On the Move: the Psychology of Change and Transition.* John Wiley & Sons, Chichester.

Ogier, M.E. (1989) *Working and Learning - the Learning Environment in Clinical Nursing.* Scutari Press, London.

Orton, H.D. (1981) *Ward Learning Climate.* RCN Research Series, Royal College of Nursing, London.

Orton, H.D. (1983) Ward learning climate and student response, in Davis, B. (ed) *Research into Nurse Education.* Croom Helm, London.

Palmer, E.A. (1987) *The Nature of the Mentor Relationship in Nursing Education.* Unpublished BEd dissertation. Polytechnic of the South Bank, London.

Palmer, E.A. (1993) *Distinguishing Between Mentors and Preceptors.* West Midlands Regional Health Authority Conference Paper, National Exhibition Centre, Birmingham.

Parsons, R., Maclean, J., Butcher, P. & Shamian, J. (1985) The staff nurse as peer educator – preceptorship on the unit. *The Canadian Nurse,* **8**, 19–20.

Piemme, J.A., Kramer, W., Tack, B.B. & Evans, J. (1987) Developing a nurse preceptor training program. *Today's OR Nurse,* **9**, 3, 24–30.

Puetz, B.E. (1992) Needs assessment: the essence of staff development programs, in Kelly, K.J. (ed) *Nursing Staff Development – Current Competence, Future Focus.* J.B. Lippincott & Co., Philadelphia.

Ramsden, P. (1992) *Learning to Teach in Higher Education.* Routledge, London.

Reed, S. & Price, J. (1991) Audit of clinical learning areas. *Nursing Times,* **87**, 27, 57–58.

Rogers, C.R. (1993) The interpersonal relationship in the facilitation of learning, in Thorpe, M., Edward, R. & Hanson, A. (eds) *Culture and Processes of Adult Learning.* Routledge/The Open University, London.

SOED (1990) *Shorter Oxford English Dictionary* based on historical principles.

Shamian, J. & Inhaber, R. (1985) The concept and practice of preceptorship in contemporary nursing: a review of the literature. *International Journal of Nursing Studies,* **22**, 2, 79–88.

Stoter, D. (1992) The culture of care. *Nursing Times,* **88**, 12, 30–31.

Tight, M. (1985) Modelling the education of adults. *Studies in the Education of Adults,* **17**, 1, 3–18.

Turnbull, E. (1983) Rewards in nursing: the case of nurse preceptors. *Journal of Nursing Administration,* **1**, 10–13.

UKCC (1990) *The Report of the Post-Registration, Education and Practice Project (PREPP report).* United Kingdom Central Council, London.

UKCC (1992) *Code of Professional Conduct* (3rd edition). United Kingdom Central Council, London.

UKCC (1993) Registrar's Letter *The Council's Position Concerning a Period of Support and Preceptorship: Implementation of the Post-Registration Education and Practice Project proposals.* January 4, United Kingdom Central Council, London.

Westra, R.J. & Graziano, M.J. (1992) Preceptors: a comparison of their perceived needs before and after the preceptor experience. *The Journal of Continuing Education in Nursing,* **23**, 5, 212–15.1

Wright, S. (1986) *Changing Nursing Practice.* Edward Arnold, London.

Zerbe, M.B. & Lachat, M.F. (1991) A three-tiered team model for undergraduate preceptor programs. *Nurse Educator,* **16**, 19–21.

Chapter 5
The Support Agenda: What's in it for the Patient?

Together with the empowerment and freedom to change offered by Project 2000, midwives, nurses and health visitors are now in an excellent position to assert themselves as expert clinical role models for all health care staff. By working with colleagues and sharing the problems and anxieties apparent in learning to carry out complex and demanding work, the time appears to have arrived for a re-working of traditional and ad hoc support systems, so that the support roles previously explored can be matched to staff working in widely varying environments and situations.

Steps needed to implement a support system

Approaches to implementation need to be viewed on both a strategic and a local level, so that everyone involved is aware of the ways in which support is to be provided, monitored and evaluated. On a wider, operational and strategic level it is necessary to:

- Formally assess where support is required.
- Determine who will provide and pay for it.
- Appoint or second staff to carry out the selection and preparation of support staff.
- Decide on the nature of support role required in a given area.
- Clarify mutual expectations for such a role.
- Allocate support roles appropriately according to locally meaningful guidelines.

On a local level it is necessary to build up good communication networks so that plans for the proposed system are understood and anticipated by staff. The co-operation of individual managers and their staff will be needed to assist in:

- Formal assessment of learning support needs.
- Setting up of a local support structure.
- Setting realistic and helpful selection criteria for staff interested in taking on a support role.
- Selecting and allocating staff.
- Planning for and seconding staff for formal role preparation.
- Dissemination of ideas and information related to the proposed system (or adaptation of existing systems).
- Working out the best ways of monitoring support systems locally.
- Developing ethical and procedural guidelines for dealing with any potentially difficult issues or problems.
- Integrating the support mechanisms into other professional areas, such as staff appraisals, career counselling and the development of professional portfolios.
- The development of user-friendly documentation as required by the support roles offered.

Determining priorities

Areas which are well-established for the purposes of teaching and learning, such as those approved by the national boards for nursing, midwifery and health visiting, are likely to have some form of support roles already in place. The allocation of students and qualified staff on course placements may mean that specific support roles are used according to the course planning team's criteria. These roles in turn may have been interpreted according to guidelines provided by course leaders, colleges, or the boards' own requirements.

Recognizing that earlier interpretations of such roles have tended to be confusing, it would seem reasonable to suggest, as a first step, a possible re-examination of the definitions and remits of each role, afresh, in the light of the conceptual clarification offered in the previous chapters on mentoring and preceptorship.

Where existing support systems are working well and staff are at ease with themselves, it would equally be of help to tease out what aspects of the provision offered are the most positive and useful, and to communicate these more fully, so that others who have had less enjoyable experiences can build on the success of colleagues, rather than merrily re-inventing the same wheels.

Our colleagues in psychiatry and the community have a distinguished history of support roles in relation to clinical supervision within their own fields (Butterworth & Faugier, 1992). In order to build on these in the context of preceptorship it is important to try (if possible) to differentiate between aspects of supervision and support in their interpretations of what is intended primarily as supervision. The balance of preceptorship would appear to lean towards support rather than supervision, but there is a need to test this thoroughly in application.

In our experience of developing both roles for clinical practice, it has become clear that the single most taxing problem for staff hoping to introduce support roles – or refine existing ones – is the need for conceptual clarity over the differences between mentoring and preceptorship.

This is often the first question asked by staff undertaking teaching and assessment courses, and the one which affords them the most anguish.

Another priority, therefore, before even considering implementation is a careful assessment of what is required and by whom. What are the issues at stake and who is best qualified to address these issues?

Given the evolving partnership between higher education and the professions, and the opportunities being offered by the new NHS culture to innovate according to local need, there would seem to be no reason why support roles cannot be introduced and developed on a shared, equal basis with service and education staff.

It is also essential to recognize and establish effective partnership arrangements between service and education to ensure that this time around, the mentoring and preceptorship learning support initiatives are understood and implemented successfully to the benefit of all concerned.

Role comparisons

What may have confused those planning the implementation of these two learning support roles in the past, is that both mentor and preceptor relationships appear to possess many of the same inherent qualities and characteristics. This would be expected as both provide enabling, supportive relationships. As can be seen from the previous chapters there are similarities in approach, which, in the past, have caused managers and educators difficulties in making a clear distinction of the two roles, causing them to be used inappropriately.

Both mentoring and preceptorship provide an enabling relationship of some intensity but the mentor relationship is one of closer, emotional intimacy. In making a comparison, both Shapiro *et al.* (1978) and Puetz (1985), identified a continuum of roles that ranged from role modelling through preceptorship to that of mentoring. This can be illustrated in Fig. 5.1 to show how the separate entities relate to each other in terms of the degree of intimacy required within the identified relationships. Until

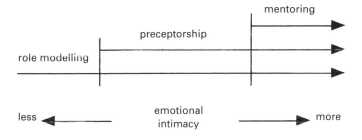

Fig. 5.1   Relationships of support roles.

these early conceptualizations of the different roles, it was relatively easy to confuse functions and to experience difficulty in appreciating where the application of role modelling might fit with the more enabling roles of mentoring and preceptorship.

Lack of clarity has also arisen because of a basic misrepresentation of the nature of the classical mentor and how, without due care and attention, it can be stripped of its essential qualities and reduced to a more simplified, functional relationship. What is important now is to recognize that the roles of mentoring and preceptorship are complementary and of equal value in providing learning support and socialization. The two roles may vary in nature, duration, context and practical application but they both have a valuable part to play in assisting in the personal development of individuals.

The differences between mentoring and preceptorship

Clarity in the nature of the differences is offered by Deane & Campbell (1985). In comparing mentor and preceptor functions they suggested that mentors took a specific, personal interest in assisting an individual practitioner with career development. This enabled the mentor to enhance career planning and encourage personal and professional satisfaction in those they were mentoring. To achieve this the mentor and mentoree had to be in regular, close contact but they did not necessarily have to be working within the same clinical setting.

In comparison, preceptors 'act as agents for their employers, to assist other employees or students in adjusting to their new role' (Deane & Campbell, 1985, p. 144). It is important that preceptors and preceptees work closely together in partnership with structured objectives, clear expectations or outcomes for a specified duration, where there is an element of formal assessment in the form of 'objective processes for measuring achievement' (Deane & Campbell, 1985, p. 144). The resulting supportive individualized teaching and learning interaction enables practitioners to develop their knowledge and skills within a trusting relationship.

Traditionally, the preceptor role in its application specifically for students, has come to represent that of the clinical practitioner who facilitates day-to-day practice, teaching and assessing while having clinical responsibilities. As previously identified in Chapter 4, this has been recently adapted by these working on the PREPP report to relate to an experienced, registered practitioner who works in partnership with a newly registered, or 'returning' qualified practitioner. The preceptor provides assistance and support in the process of learning and adaptation to their new roles (Morton-Cooper, 1991). This fits well with the notion of preceptorship as suggested by Deane & Campbell (1985).

Mentoring is more personally directed to assist in setting a wider exposure to the world of work. The preceptor, in contrast, assists with practice development and clinical competence. The mentor may also assist with practical concerns at certain points in the duration of the relationship, but essentially the mentor is more concerned with professional development in terms of broader career issues.

A preceptor assists in the socialization process but, once again, the role as it presents will be functional and related more specifically to the clinical environment. In preceptorship the emphasis is on working towards the mutually agreed and established goals and outcomes. The mentor, by comparison, widens an individual's personal network and assists with the social and professional introductions within the larger arena of professional practice.

Classical mentoring is determined by the natural pairing of the partnership to provide unstructured learning support. In preceptorship the basis for the relationship is that of structured learning support. This structure is determined by the requirements of the profession and the organization, framed within specified or structured outcomes which, of course, can and should be negotiated and mutually agreed.

In terms of the specified outcomes, some programmes of formal mentoring with identified outcomes and an over-reliance on structure, will blur the boundaries between the two roles as can be seen in Figure 5.2. This diagram is adapted from Fig. 3.4 to show the possible boundaries of both mentoring and preceptorship as applied to clinical practice. The continuum illustrates the range of approaches from classical mentoring through semi-structured formats, to that of more structured applications of formal mentoring.

Exploring this continuum aids in setting the artificial boundaries between mentoring and preceptorship. The diagram demonstrates where mentoring – in its formal application to health care, with the assignment of contract mentors – crosses the boundary of that of the

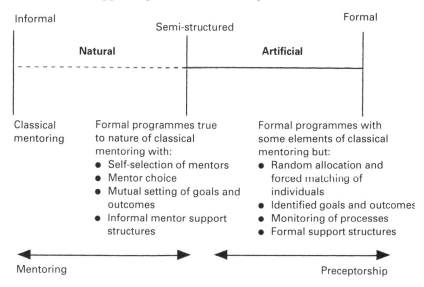

Fig. 5.2 The continuum of informality and formality, classical mentoring, formal mentoring, and preceptorship.

more clinically orientated, preceptor role. It becomes easier to appreciate how, in recent years, confusion arose as formal mentoring approaches were put into practice and preceptorship programmes developed. Classical mentoring is naturally determined by the individuals who enter into the relationship. Once mentoring programmes are constructed that have formally identified set outcomes, monitoring elements, reliance on preparation as 'training for mentors', and approved support structures, the boundaries between the two roles become decidedly less distinct.

Much evidence, both empirical and anecdotal, demonstrates the long-term nature of classical mentoring relationships. The mentor has broader responsibilities for assisting in the personal and career development of those they are in partnership with. The complex and dynamic nature of the collaboration is dependent upon the personal characteristics of each of the partners to sustain it through the peaks and troughs of a long-term, essentially adaptive, relationship. As has been previously discussed, the duration of the relationship is set by the collaborating individuals. For the mentoring process to be initiated and developed to its full potential, anything between two and fifteen years provides the expected lifespan for such relationships. This is in direct contrast to the newly formulated ideas about preceptorship programmes in nursing, midwifery and health visiting which are much more practice-based,

Table 5.1 Overview of differences between mentoring and preceptorship.

Mentor	Preceptor
Intimate, personal enabling relationship	Functional enabling relationship
Career socialization, providing social and political networks	Clinical socialization in initial post-registration period
Unstructured learning support	Structured learning support
Longer duration	Short duration, related to clinical allocation ⁙ᵖᵉᶜⁱᶠⁱᶜ ᵖᵉʳⁱᵒᵈ ᵒᶠ ˢᵘᵖᵖᵒʳᵗ
Multi-faceted roles but no formal assessment	Specific roles with emphasis on teaching, role modelling and assessment as performance evaluation
Chosen by individual	Chosen by employer/staff development/ continuing education staff

employer- or professionally-directed with a predetermined 'shelf life' of four months.

In cases of classical mentoring the practitioners select each other, as previously stated. In formal mentoring, selection or assigning of mentors may occur but in preceptorship it appears likely that individuals will be identified and paired together for the duration of the specified programme of development.

A summary of the differences between mentoring and preceptorship is presented in Table 5.1. Here, the differences between the two support roles are clearly shown in terms of their nature, function and duration.

In beginning to tease out the differences between these two complex support roles, it is easy to see why, in the past, such difficulties were experienced. What is important now is that we acknowledge the mistakes of the past and work positively to ensure that each of these enabling roles are given the recognition that it deserves.

A basis for partnership

The need for support which resounds in the British literature (see Morton-Cooper (1992) for a literature review) is a strong argument for college staff to work together with service managers and in-service support staff, to bring together the strengths and skills of both in the spirit of colleagueship. The support and leadership of regional health authority staff can also be a tremendous impetus for innovation.

Models of professional education developed could then be sensitive to the pressures affecting the workplace, and the theoretical concepts advocated by teaching staff who have the requisite background and expertise in education; such a combination allows for learners' progress to be monitored and feedback given as appropriate to the level and demands of any course or period of career transition.

The development of nursing support teams, such as that at Dudley Road Hospital, Birmingham, has been instrumental in helping clinical and managerial staff to re-appraise existing clinical learning environments, question current limitations, and reassess the prevailing philosophies of care offered to patients on a day-to-day basis. The fertile ground of NHS and professional reforms has led to significant shifts in the way staff are expected to carry out their work – particularly with regard to role development, resource management, standards of care, clinical competencies expected of staff working at different grades, and, ultimately, any progression towards advanced practice.

It has to be recognized, however, that limited financial and staffing resources can place severe time constraints on staff hoping to enact change. However enthusiastic or willing staff are to help, someone needs to keep an overview on which resources are the most cost-effective in human as well as financial terms.

Appropriate delegation of roles and the need to express fears and worries about the possible implications of change are an essential part of the coping process. Ogier has pointed out that the raising of staff's awareness as to how care *should* be can arouse distress when they feel that such standards are not always being met (Ogier, 1989).

The starting point for the delivery of support is a feeling of empathy and trust, and of mutual understanding between employer and employee. Before exposing ourselves to a re-appraisal of the status quo, then, it is necessary to establish a feeling of trust and mutual respect in a team or between colleagues working closely together. Because some staff work directly with clients and have only minimal contact with other team members, extra effort should be made to provide a forum for support which enables lone professionals (for example, community staff working in rural areas) to meet on a regular basis with at least one individual who understands and has some experience of the work they undertake.

The apparent priorities for implementing support are:

- Establishing the policy and procedural steps necessary for the re-appraisal of current support systems;
- Establishing a basis for partnership with service and education colleagues;

- Re-affirming the trust and respect offered to and between colleagues in the work situation;
- Providing a forum for support which allows for uncertainties to be expressed calmly and clearly;
- Accepting the need to explore mutual understanding of support roles and to clarify these for any future use.

Issues of quality in learning support: an overview of ethical concepts

There are certain fundamental questions to be asked when considering the quality of learning support offered to students and staff:

- Is the support accessible?
- Do staff know who to turn to for help and advice?
- Are the intentions of support offered clear and unambiguous?
- Is any formal support process explained fully in advance and opportunities offered for questions and clarification?
- How user-friendly is the documentation associated with support? (e.g. evaluation methods, learning contracts, critical incident reports, ethical guidelines) Is this easily referred to and yet confidential of its sources? (By common consent, confidentiality is an important element in nursing (Brown, Kitson & McKnight, 1992). Patients and clients expect it and so do staff.)

Katz has looked at the developmental career stages of teachers and described them as *survival, consolidation, renewal* and *maturity* (see Katz, cited in Cervero, 1988). Given that nurses also work within a service profession it is possible to see direct comparisons between such stages.

A period of transition is likely to follow each stage, with elements of all four stages entering into a person's coping strategy at each stage. Therefore, it is necessary when providing a support system to be sensitive to the issues and personalities involved. Sensitivity to a person's self-image and work identity is vital, as work identities operate as both causes and consequences of (women's) work lives, and stand in systematic relation to other aspects of their lives, such as schooling and family (Rosenfeld & Spenner, 1988).

The support system that fails to identify the self-image of its clients and work towards positive reinforcement may not help learners to participate fully in its goals. We need to analyse the factors that both motivate and *de*motivate learners so that strategies can be developed to meet the constraints these produce.

Some staff will consider their work identities and roles extremely important, while others will see them as less significant, and therefore less worthy of spending intensive time and effort on. Bevis (1988) (in Leddy & Pepper, 1989) lists the following as effective motivating strategies for learning. They would make a sound basis for an evaluation of any learning support programme provided:

- Engage the learner in active analysis
- Raise questions
- Nurture the learner
- Nurture the ethical ideal
- Nurture the caring role
- Nurture the creative drive
- Nurture curiosity and the search for satisfying ideas
- Nurture assertiveness
- Nurture the desire to seek dialogue

(see Leddy & Pepper, 1989, p. 331)

Just as we seek to develop standards of care for patients, standards of support should be developed which reflect the currency of therapeutic role models in nursing, midwifery and health visiting.

Therapeutic nursing is nursing that deliberately achieves beneficial outcomes with patients (McMahon, 1991). McMahon (1991) identified six therapeutic activities in nursing, all of which, it could be argued, could usefully be included in the implementation of staff support roles in clinical practice. These are:

(1) Developing partnership, intimacy and reciprocity in the nursing relationship.
(2) Manipulating the environment.
(3) Teaching.
(4) Providing comfort.
(5) Adopting complementary health practices.
(6) Utilizing tested physical interventions.

Taking the latter three activities literally, there is no reason why, in addition to formal support relationships, relaxation therapies and good, plain friendship can't be a major contributor to the development of a positive and conducive learning atmosphere. The power of laughter and a sense of humour to diffuse tension and regain perspective is well-recognized in the management of stressful and awkward situations (Nash, 1988).

What's in it for the patient?

As Smith has found in her study of nurses' 'caring trajectories', the styles and strategies nurses adopt in order to cope are an important facet of their ability to give and receive care (Smith, 1992). The potency of negative stereotyping and over-classification of people is a major determinant in the quality of care received by patients in every care setting (Moss, 1988).

Moss argues that nursing is a profession which readily lends itself to the rapid formation of attitudes towards those who come into contact with it, with common subdivisions or categorizations being diagnosis, or labelling of 'awkward' or 'difficult' patients. It isn't hard to find examples of stereotyping of learners as difficult, stupid or lazy, disinterested, overzealous, and so on.

Whether this is a fair or accurate analysis of nurses' attitudes generally is not known for sure, but certainly by learning to respect one another as colleagues and professionals it is possible that we might begin to elicit the reasons behind certain kinds of negative or aggressive behaviours in students or staff, and thus begin to perceive how patients and clients feel to be on the receiving end of the same kind of stereotyping.

Smith (1992) identified the distancing strategies employed by senior staff who found themselves unable to deal with embarrassing and difficult situations, and therefore unsympathetic to the needs of students and more junior staff:

> '... these included distancing strategies such as developing a "seen it all before attitude" which made it easier to label patients and their behaviour. Thus by slotting patients into convenient categories such as "difficult", "awkward", "a pain", or a "nuisance", and projecting images and assumptions upon them associated with their gender, class and race, ... nurses were able to "objectify" them and their symptoms'.

> (Smith, 1991, p. 131)

Support is about not having to objectify fellow human beings, and about responding to them in a natural and sincere way. But that isn't to say that people don't test us out sometimes!

The concept of caring is central to nursing and to role-modelling. Nelms *et al.* (1993) asked the following questions in a research study:

- Do students learn about caring from observing role- modelling in classroom and clinical settings?
- How do students' experiences of caring and non-caring in a nursing curriculum influence what they learn about caring?

Both of these questions are central to the thesis of support via mentoring and preceptorship, and bring the issue of care for patients and care for colleagues directly together. The hypotheses generated from their study revealed that there are a variety of relationships through which students experience and learn about caring.

Their relationships with others helped them to value the potential for caring with families and patients. Self-awareness of caring opportunities was all-important, and the authors of the study reminded staff and college tutors to be aware of the 'gaze' upon us as we strive to be authentic models for students and staff.

In promoting effective role-models for staff development we do need to clarify roles and approaches, and apply these to an appropriate context. It is pointless re-enacting the mistakes of the past and merely transferring a superficial or inadequately perceived role on to a member of staff who has no authoritative help or personal and professional support network to tap into.

This would be the same as sending a patient to theatre and forgetting to collect him; asking a parent to monitor a child's diabetes and neglecting to educate him about what to do; assisting a young person with learning difficulties into a home of his own, without being there through some of the hard times!

Providing support for continuing learning in the health professions is concerned with the quality of educational and work experience we would all like to share. Promoting a sense of common goals and identity, a sense of holism, a sense of 'being there' for each other and, ultimately, for our patients.

Although changing and enriching the culture of nursing will be a lifetime's venture for most of us, it is important not to lose sight of what is important to us. Nelms *et al.* express it perfectly in a single paragraph:

'The secret, we believe, is related to teaching caring encounters of an ethical kind, perhaps even a type of love, not of the romantic kind, but a learning entanglement in which admiration for the knowledge and competence of a caring expert, curiosity about the subject matter of our discipline, and feelings of amazement and excitement are evoked in the learner throughout the process of acquiring knowledge and skills'.

(Nelms, Jones & Gray, 1993, p. 23)

This book has attempted to convey such sentiments through the constructive development, adaptation and refinement of support roles within practice, supported by educational theory and conceptual analysis. By stimulating and sharing in the debate, our endeavours have been to clarify the complexities of support in clinical practice. What matters now is that the dialogue continues, and support in action becomes a meaningful, practical reality.

References

Brown, J.M., Kitson, A.L. & McKnight, T.J. (1992) *Challenges in Caring: Explorations in Nursing and Ethics.* Chapman and Hall, London.

Butterworth, T. & Faugier, J. (Eds) 1992) *Clinical Supervision and Mentorship in Nursing.* Chapman and Hall, London.

Cervero, R.M. (1988) *Effective Continuing Education for Professionals.* Jossey Bass, London.

Deane, D. & Campbell, J. (1985) *Developing Professional Effectiveness in Nursing.* Reston Publications, Virginia.

Leddy, S. & Pepper, J.M. (1989) *Conceptual Bases of Professional Nursing.* J.B. Lippincott & Co, Philadelphia.

McMahon, R. & Pearson, A. (1991) *Nursing as Therapy.* Chapman and Hall, London.

Morton-Cooper, A. (1992) *An Evaluation of Preceptorship as an Appropriate Conceptual Model for British Continuing Nurse Education,* MEd dissertation, University of Warwick.

Morton-Cooper, A. (1993) *Expectations of the Preceptor Relationship.* West Midlands Regional Health Authority Conference Paper, National Exhibition Centre, Birmingham.

Moss, A.R. (1988) Determinants of patient care: nursing process or nursing attitudes? *Journal of Advanced Nursing,* **13**, 615–20.

Nash, W. (1988) *At Ease with Stress – the Approach of Wholeness.* Darton, Longman and Todd, London.

Nelms, T.P., Jones, J.M. & Gray, D.P. (1993) Role modelling: a method for teaching caring in nursing education. *Journal of Nursing Education,* **32**, 1, 18–23.

Ogier, M. (1989) *Working and Learning.* Scutari Press, London.

Puetz, B.E. (1985) Learn the ropes from a mentor. *Nursing Success Today*, **2**, 6, 11–13.

Rosenfeld, R.A. & Spenner, K.I. (1988) Women's work and women's careers – a dynamic analysis of work identity in the early life course, in White Riley, M. (ed) *Social Structure and Human Lives.*

Shapiro, E.C., Hascltinc, F. & Rowe, M. (1978) Moving up: role models, mentors and the patron system. *Sloan Management Review*, **19**, 51–8.

Smith, P. (1992) *The Emotional Labour of Nursing.* McMillan, Basingstoke.

Postscript

Reginald H. Pyne
OBE, RGN, RFN, FBIM
Assistant Registrar, Standards and Ethics
United Kingdom Central Council for Nursing, Midwifery and
Health Visiting

My first thought on completing my reading of the Preface and 5 chapters of this text in order to respond to the invitation to write a Postscript were that such further labour on my part was unnecessary. The basis for this reaction was the fact that I regarded the work as having been done in the first few paragraphs of the Preface and the last few paragraphs of the final chapter.

The former passage of text rightly and accurately emphasizes the need to address the difficulties faced by staff who need to continue to learn in the workplace. It also emphasizes that all nursing staff in practice settings who have any responsibility for the development and teaching of staff should heed the messages which the book goes on to present. The latter passage of text presents the reader with the essential question of 'What's in it for the patient?', and concludes with an unequivocal challenge to the profession to satisfy the expectations the book has clearly presented.

My second thoughts might possibly be regarded by the reader as in conflict with my first thought, for these were that much of the text that I had read (and enjoyed reading) was a compilation of statements of the obvious. I hasten to add that for me to think such thoughts must not be taken by the reader as implying that I think this text was unnecessary and should not have been written. Quite the reverse is true. After all, as a senior officer of the United Kingdom Central Council for Nursing, Midwifery and Health Visiting I have been party to the preparation, publication and distribution of a number of extremely important documents, much of the contents of which were also statements of the obvious. *The Scope of Professional Practice* (1992), not referred to in this text, but clearly relevant to its important themes, is one such publication. What is – or should be – obvious sometimes needs to be said repeatedly.

I have referred to the opening and closing sequences of the text as possibly rendering my task redundant. Between those passages, however, I find a wide range of important and relevant issues addressed.

How pleasing it is to find a text which recognizes the difficulties involved in the transition from lay person to confident and competent registered nurse. How pleasing it is to find such a rejection of the all too common impression given by established practitioners that this transition happens as if by magic and without harm or risk to those who, at times of great vulnerability, dependence and anxiety, require the services of nurses.

Confident, competent and effective practice has many component parts and many facets. The authors are right to reject the implication that those new to the profession of nursing should prove themselves by '... sailing the same waters and overcoming the same fears in the same haphazard and unnecessarily painful ways'.

I have not regarded my role in writing this Postscript as to re-state the main arguments that have been developed so cogently by the authors in a clearly referenced text. I do choose, however, to draw attention to and underline certain issues which might not have been regarded by the reader as central to the subject of the book but which I do regard in that light.

Impressions, words and phrases that are scattered throughout the text cluster together in my mind and, together, become inseparable from the main subject and the context in which it must be considered. Reference to 'subservience' is there, and necessarily so since, in spite of encouragement to change emanating from the profession's statutory regulatory body, and opportunities to change arising, too many remain prepared to accept a subservient or passively submissive role.

Reference can also be found to freedom and responsibility, autonomy and judgement and to the need for practitioners who have the capacity to be self-directing.

These things, important though they are, cannot be achieved and enjoyed, and the resulting benefits cannot be made available to patients unless we assist students, newly registered practitioners, those who move to a different area of professional practice and those returning to practice after a break to cross the bridge, make the required transition and quickly achieve the levels of confidence and competence required. This is also the route to the personal enrichment that derives from genuine job satisfaction.

The promotion of an approach which is enabling rather than disabling and which can develop quickly the scope of practice of an individual practitioner commands my support.

Never more than now has there been a need for good and effective role models. Far from being regarded as a questionable feature of a market orientated system of health care provision, or as something that has to be fought for and justified, I contend that the possession of such role models and a system in which they can operate effectively should be regarded by a provider as a marketing asset. It should be seen in this light for the simple reason that it is declaring that the provider has a genuine interest in the best possible outcome for the person who has no option but to become a patient.

This book, by examining what might be seen as a narrow subject in a wide-ranging and imaginative way, by closing with a challenge to the profession to satisfy its high expectations, and by addressing openly the problems and difficulties of the context in which practitioners practise, has the potential to contribute to improvement in the care of patients. Whether that potential becomes a reality is, in large part, in your hands, dear reader.

Index

academic adviser
  mature students, 41
  roles and responsibilities, 41–2, 43
adult learning, 8, 16, 58–9
  diagnosing, 12
  processes, 6, 11, 13, 20
  reflectivity, 12–13
  typology, 17–18
assessment, 122–3, 149
  learning needs, 129
  peer, 122
  preceptor, 123
assessor(s), 123

benefits
  mentoring, 75
  preceptorship, 106, 108–109
burnout, 105

case studies
  mentoring, 87–94
  issues, 91
changing work cultures, 29–30
classical mentoring, see mentoring
clinical audit, 132
clinical instructor(s), 101, 108
clinical learning environments, 5
clinical resource file, 137
  adult education, 139
  assessment, 141
  budgeting, costing and planning in
    new NHS, 138
  clinical education communication
    skills, 138
  contract learning, 141

counselling and support skills, 141
  critical incident analysis, 141
  personal management skills, 139
  philosophical theories of education,
    139
  preceptorships and nursing staff
    development, 140
  professional education, 139
  profiling and career planning, 141
  psychology, 141
  role theory and analysis, 141
clinical supervisor(s), 40
  supervision, 43–4, 147
clinical teaching, 2
coach, 47–8, 63
  facilitator, 46–7
coaching functions, 47–8, 63
collaborative relationships, 100
colleagueship, 137, 152
conflict
  role, 135
  value, 103–104
continuing professional education, see
    education, continuing
contract
  learning, 107, 131
  mentor, 38
  mentoring, 150–51
counsellor
  mentoring, 63, 68
critical reflection, see reflection
cross gender mentoring, 92
culture
  definition, 65
  organizational, 65–6
curriculum, see programme

disablers, 52
    toxic mentors, 50–51
disabling traits, 49–50
distinguishing between
    mentors and preceptors, 149–52

education
    continuing, 13–15, 38, 102, 130–31
    in-service, 10–11, 101
    mentor in initial teacher training, 85
    mentoring, 87–8
    of equals, 24–5
    relationships, 100
emotional
    phases, 36
    support, 35–6
emotions, 35–6
enabler(s), 52, 133
enabling, 49–52, 148–9, 152
    traits, 52
evaluation
    mentor programmes, 86
    preceptor programmes, 110–12, 128,
        131–2
experiential learning, 19–21, 134
    cycle, 19
    taxonomies, 21

facilitated mentoring, *see* contract
    mentoring
facilitation, 21, 44–5, 51, 135
facilitator(s), 45
    coach, 46–7
    key functions, 48–9
    resource, 64
    roles and responsibilities, 47
feedback, 47–8
Fordism, 29
formal mentoring, *see* contract
    mentoring

growth and development, 23, 49, 57–9,
    62, 105
guide/networker, 63

Health Service changes, 30–32, 153

higher education, 41–3, 44, 148

internal market, 31

learning
    adult, 6
    agenda, 16, 47
    audit, 132
    contract, 107, 131
    climate, 131
    culture, 9 10, 88
    environments, 4–5, 129–32
    experiential, 19–21, 134
    humanist approaches, 20–21
    motivation strategies, 155
    needs analysis, 129–33
    open learning, 18
    opportunities, 20–21
    process, 5
    reflectivity, 12–13
    situations, 5
    society, 9–10
    support, 34–35

mature students, 41
mentor
    characteristics/qualities, 72–4
    classical, *see* mentoring
    contract, 38, 65–6, 77, 150
    definition(s), 57, 60, 62
    helper functions, 62–4
    history/origins, 57
    influences, 58
    labels, 58
    midwifery, 69, 87, 92
    pool, 67, 83
    role, 61–4
    selection, 82
    signal, 61
    support, 86
    toxic, 50–51, 75–6
mentor programmes, 77, 81–5
    aims/outcomes, 84
    evaluation, 86
    initial teacher training, 68, 85
    preparation, 81

mentoree
  matching, 83–4
  qualities, 74–5
mentoring
  adviser, 62–3
  approaches, 68
  business, 67
  case studies, 87–94
  classical, 38, 61–8, 93–4, 149–52
  challenges, 60
  constraints, 76–7
  cross gender, 92
  definition(s), 59, 61
  formal, *see* contract, mentor
  influences, 58–9
  language/terms, 57–8, 65–7
  limitations, 75–7
  origins/history, 57
  phases, 70–72
  preceptorship differences, 149–52
  pseudo/quasi, 66–7
  true, *see* classical
mentorship, *see* mentoring

network(er), 38, 63
  social, 38, 40–41, 136–7
nurse
  case study, 87–8
  clinical supervision, 43–4
  educator(s), 9, 12
  expert, 112–13
  image, 2–3
  primary, 118
  training, 8–9

occupational therapy, 68
  case study, 89–91, 93–4

partnership(s), 152–3
  collaborative, 65
patient(s), 146, 155–6
peer(s)
  group, 40–41
  support, 111–12, 113
personal tutor(s)
  role/responsibilities, 42–3

physiotherapy, 68
  case study, 88–9, 92–3
post Fordism/postmodernism, 29–30
preceptor
  accountability, 126
  assessment, 122–3
  attributes, 109
  definition (UK), 103
  definitions, 100–102
  designated, 127–8
  learning needs, 129–32
  outcomes, 122
  preparation, 108, 111, 118–122,
    129–31
  qualities, 106
  role/responsibilities, 38, 99–100, 106,
    150
  selection, 105, 111, 118
  student tryad, 108
  support, 111, 131
  unit, 127–8
  workshops, 129
preceptorship
  accountability, 126
  American interpretations, 100,
    102–109
  benefits, 106, 108–109
  descriptions, 99–100
  evaluation, 110, 112, 128
  in nursing, 101
  mentoring differences, 149–52
  model for practice, 125–9
  relationship expectations, 110–13
  UKCC guidelines, 102, 113–18
primary practice
  UK interpretations, 115, 118
programme
  interpretations, 124
  medical, 3
  model, 124–5
  model for preceptorship, 125–9,
    134–5, 138
Project 2000, 19, 42–4, 146
pseudo/quasi mentoring, 66–7
psychology of transition, 135

qualified, 37–8, 99–100
quasi mentoring, 66–7

reality shock, 110, 113
reflection, 5, 12, 14, 16, 34–35, 47–48,
　　131, 137
reflectivity, 12–13
relationships, 38
　collaborative, 38, 100, 137
　peer, 40–41
　supervisory, *see* supervision
resources
　facilitator, 64
　mentor programmes, 80
role
　change, 16
　comparisons, 148–152
　modelling, 62–63
　models, 24, 157
　theory, 135

safe space, 136–137
selection
　mentorees, 83
　mentors, 82
　preceptors, 105, 118
self awareness, 59, 64
　discovery, 59
shared learning opportunities, 3
skilled helper, 35–6, 137
social
　support, 136–7
　work supervision, 44
socialization, 43, 105, 110, 150
　mentoring, 59
sponsor(ship)
　business, 67
　mentoring, 63
　nursing, 104
staff development, 16, 38, 73, 80,
　　125–6, 138, 157
status passage, 3
strategies
　coping, 156
　distancing, 156

enabling and disabling, 49–52
　motivation, 155
student
　mature, 41
　services, 43
　see supervision/support
stress overload, 22–3
supervision
　authoritarian, 46
　nursing, 43–4
　professional, 11, 117
　student, 4, 43–4
supervisors
　clinical, 40, 43, 47
　mental health, 44
　midwifery, 44
supervisory relationships, *see*
　　supervisors
support
　academic advisors, 41–2
　emotional, 35–6
　frameworks, 31, 33, 37–8
　implementation, 146–8, 153–4
　learning, 34–5
　mentor, 86
　pastoral, 42
　personal tutors, 43
　preceptor, 111
　quality, 154
　roles, 39–43, 45–8
　selection criteria, 49
　students, 37–40, 38–49
　systems, 33–4, 146–8

teacher(s)
　case study, 89, 93
　developmental career stages, 154
　initial training, 85
　mentoring, 64
theory practice gap, 19, 47–8, 102–103,
　　106
therapeutic nursing, 155
toxic mentors, 50–51, 75–6
transition cycle, 135
　psychology, 135

trusts
  self governing, 31, 33
  new relationships, 31, 32–3
tutor(s)
  personal, 42–3
  see academic adviser
typology of adult learners, 17

United Kingdom Central Council
    (UKCC), 25, 38, 42–4, 107, 108,
    111, 113–18, 120, 121–2

virtual world, 48

work based learning support, 68